Wanessa Silva Garcia Medina

Aromatic Anticonvulsants and their effects on mitochondrial function

Wanessa Silva Garcia Medina

Aromatic Anticonvulsants and their effects on mitochondrial function

Carbamazepine, Phenytoin and Phenobarbital and their areno-oxides on mitochondrial function and oxidative stress

ScienciaScripts

Imprint

Cover image: www.ingimage.com

This book is a translation from the original published under ISBN 978-3-330-77214-4.

Publisher:
Sciencia Scripts
is a trademark of
Dodo Books Indian Ocean Ltd. and OmniScriptum S.R.L publishing group

120 High Road, East Finchley, London, N2 9ED, United Kingdom
Str. Armeneasca 28/1, office 1, Chisinau MD-2012, Republic of Moldova, Europe
Managing Directors: Ieva Konstantinova, Victoria Ursu
info@omniscriptum.com

Printed at: see last page
ISBN: 978-620-8-64103-0

SUMMARY

DEDICATORY

I dedicate this step to my parents, my grandmother, my children and my husband, for the trust and encouragement they have always given me and I hope that this step will bear good fruit and serve as a good example for my children.

THANKS

- I would like to thank Dr. Antonio Cardozo dos Santos (my advisor) for the opportunity to do my doctorate with a competent and reliable professional, who was always there to guide me and help me at every stage of my doctorate, just as he did during my master's degree;
- Dr. Neife Aparecida Guinaim dos Santos, for helping me to complete this stage and always being willing to collaborate throughout the process;
- I'm very grateful for always having the love, friendship, companionship and loyalty of my sister Fabiola, who has helped me a lot over the years, constantly collaborating on bureaucratic issues and always encouraging me, giving me good advice on the direction I should take in my professional life;
- I am very grateful to my parents, who for almost 32 years have encouraged my cultural and personal development, giving me the chance to become a better person with a different culture;
- To my husband Evandro Marcio Medina, for his understanding and consent, for my absence during some periods of our lives, because we were physically separated, so that I could do my doctorate, for the moments that we stopped sharing in order to build a good that we believe is important for us and our children;
- To Natalino Bocardo, who was there every step of the way and was always an excellent friend, and to the staff of the Biochemistry laboratory, for the kindness with which they always treated me and for always being helpful.
- To Professor Dr. Maria Vitória Bentley, for her friendship and trust, making it possible for me to grow in my research.

SUMMARY

The liver plays a central role in the metabolic disposal of various endogenous and exogenous chemical agents, including almost all drugs. This biotransformation process can lead to the formation of highly reactive intermediate metabolites which, if not properly eliminated, can interact with cellular macromolecules, damaging the organ. The idiosyncratic hepatotoxicity associated with the use of aromatic antiepileptics (AEA) is well known and has been attributed to the accumulation of toxic intermediates (areno-oxides) formed during hepatic bioactivation. Although the participation of immunological processes in the mechanism of toxic action of AEA has been demonstrated, there is the possibility of adjuvant mechanisms involving mitochondrial toxicity, an event not yet explored in the scientific literature. This study evaluated, *in vitro*, the effect of the AEA: carbamazepine, phenytoin and phenobarbital, as well as their respective metabolites on mitochondrial function and the induction of oxidative stress in rat liver mitochondria, as a possible mechanism of the hepatotoxic action of these drugs. A rat liver microsomal system was used to bioactivate the drugs and produce their metabolites *in vitro.* Without bioactivation, only phenobarbital (at high concentrations) showed inhibitory effects on state 3 respiration, ATP synthesis and membrane potential, without, however, inducing oxidative stress. When bioactivated, all the drugs showed effects on mitochondrial function through a process mediated by oxidative stress. All the bioactivated drugs affected mitochondrial respiration, causing a decrease in oxygen consumption in state 3, a decrease in RCR and an increase in oxygen consumption in state 4. Alterations in calcium uptake/release, inhibition of ATP synthesis, a decrease in membrane potential and inhibition of calcium-induced mitochondrial swelling were also evident. The oxidation of mitochondrial proteins and lipids was demonstrated by the formation of carbonylated proteins, a decrease in proteins with sulfhydryl groups, an increase in malondialdehyde (MDA) and the oxidation of cardiolipin. The mitochondrial antioxidant defense system was also affected, as evidenced by the decrease in the GSH/GSSG (reduced glutathione/oxidized glutathione) ratio. The results strongly suggest the involvement of mitochondrial damage, mediated by oxidative stress caused by the metabolites of AEA, in the development of idiosyncratic hepatotoxicity induced by these drugs.

Keywords: phenobarbital; carbamazepine; phenytoin; mitochondria; oxidative stress; hepatotoxicity; areno-oxides; aromatic antiepileptics (AEA)

INTRODUCTION

In drug development, we sometimes find changes in hepatocytes, such as steatosis, which are not accompanied by degenerative changes in the liver in non-clinical toxicity studies. Some studies have investigated the relationship between changes in hepatocytes observed in non-clinical toxicity studies of certain compounds and mitochondrial dysfunction in order to estimate the potential risk of compounds inducing drug-induced liver damage in humans[1].

Interest in drug-induced liver injury has increased dramatically in the last decade, and it has become a relevant topic for clinicians, academics, pharmaceutical companies and regulatory bodies. By investigating the current state of the art, the latest scientific findings, controversies and guidelines, we keep trying to answer the question: Do we know everything? Since the first descriptions of hepatotoxicity more than 70 years ago, more than 1000 drugs have been identified to date, yet much of our knowledge of pathophysiological principles and diagnosis remains unchanged. Clinically ranging from asymptomatic to acute or chronic hepatitis, acute liver failure, drug-induced liver injury remains one of the main causes of emerging liver transplantation. The consumption of unregulated herbal and dietary supplements has introduced new challenges in epidemiological assessment and clinical management. Numerous registries have been created, including the US Drug Induced Liver Injury Network, to further our understanding of all aspects of drug-induced liver injury. The launch of LiverTox and other online hepatotoxicity resources are used to raise awareness of drug-induced liver injury. In 2013, the first guidelines for the diagnosis and management of drug-induced liver injury were offered by the Practice Parameters Committee of the American College of Gastroenterology and together with the identification of risk factors and predictors of injury, new mechanisms of injury, refined causality assessment tools and targeted treatment options, have come to define the current state of the art, however, gaps in our knowledge still undoubtedly remain[2].

Liver damage represents a potential complication for any prescription drug, since the liver is the central organ for the metabolic disposal of practically all drugs and xenobiotics[3-5]. Many xenobiotics are biotransformed and eliminated by the liver, mainly in the form of conjugates, without this process causing any liver damage. However, some xenobiotics are concentrated to toxic levels, while others are bioactivated to intermediate reactants that can damage the liver in various ways, including inducing cancer[6-9].

Although the exact mechanism of drug-induced liver damage has not yet been delineated, two pathways seem to be involved: direct hepatotoxicity and adverse immune reactions. Most of the time, such liver damage is initiated by the bioactivation of drugs to chemically reactive metabolites, which can interact with macromolecules such as proteins, lipids and nucleic acids, resulting in protein dysfunction, DNA damage, lipoperoxidation and oxidative stress[10]. In addition, these reactive metabolites can induce disturbances in the ion gradient and intracellular calcium concentration, resulting in mitochondrial dysfunction and decreased energy production. This cellular dysfunction can culminate in hepatocellular death and possibly liver failure[11].

Among the factors that contribute to the accumulation of toxins in hepatocytes are (1) genetic alterations in enzyme systems, leading to the formation and/or accumulation of reactive metabolites; (2) competition with other drugs and (3) depletion of metabolite detoxification systems[12,13].

Since hepatocytes are the main metabolic centers of the liver, many adverse reactions can lead to their death. The most common reaction leading to cell death is the formation of covalent bonds between the metabolic reactant and biological macromolecules. Oxidation reactions can also produce electrophilic compounds or oxygen intermediates (such as superoxide anion and other free radicals) that damage cellular components[14,15].

In addition to hepatocytes, hepatotoxic agents can affect other structures in the liver. Some substances damage the bile ducts or canaliculi, causing cholestasis without significant damage to the hepatocytes. Other substances affect sinusoidal or endothelial cells, resulting in veno-occlusive disease or fibrosis, steatosis of Ito cells or even generalized damage. Liver damage can thus be classified as hepatocellular, cholestatic or mixed[16]. Mixed liver lesions include clinical manifestations of hepatocellular and cholestatic lesions[17]. Table 1 summarizes the most frequent types of damage induced in the liver as a result of the action of different xenobiotics.

LIVER DAMAGE	**AGENTS**
Direct hepatocellular damage	acetaminophen (paracetamol), carbon tetrachloride
Steatohepatitis	ethanol, tamoxifen
Idiosyncratic reaction	isoniazid, halothane, valproic acid, **antiepileptics aromatic (e.g: carbamazepine, phenobarbital, phenytoin)**
Cholestasis	Chlorpromazine, cyclosporine A, estradiol.
Granulomatous reaction	Diltiazem, quinidine, phenytoin, procainimide.
Chronic hepatitis	Nitrofurantoin, methyldopa, isoniazid, trazodone.

Table 1. Common types of drug-induced liver damage[18] .

Microvesicular steatosis	Tetracyclines, aspirin, zidovudine, didanosine, fialuridine.
Fibrosis or Cirrhosis	Metrotrexate, vitamin A, methyldopa.
Veno-occlusive disease	Cyclophosphamide
Ischemic injury	Cocaine, nicotinic acid.

Aromatic Antiepileptics (AEA) and Idiosyncratic Hepatotoxicity

Classical antiepileptics (AE) have been used extensively in the treatment of epilepsy, one of the most frequent disorders of the central nervous system, which affects approximately 1.5% of the world's population[19].

Currently, the use of LA is not restricted to the treatment of epilepsy. These drugs are also widely used in a broad spectrum of neurological and psychiatric disorders[20]. There have been many recent studies suggesting that EDs have anxiolytic properties and could therefore be an alternative treatment for anxiety disorders[2]1. AEs are also used in the treatment of neuropathic pain[22], and carbamazepine is still the drug of choice in the treatment of trigeminal neuralgia[23].

Idiosyncratic hepatotoxicity is a well-known complication associated with AE treatment[24]. It can occur as an isolated event or as part of a multiple disorder, characterized by fever, skin rashes, eosinophilia, atypical lymphocytosis, arthralgia, lymphadenopathy, with the involvement of several organs, including the liver (hepatitis)[25]. Idiosyncratic reactions associated with the use of AE are rare but potentially fatal and have been most commonly reported with the use of aromatic antiepileptics (AEA), such as phenytoin, carbamazepine and phenobarbital[26]. The effects of aromatic anticonvulsants on the liver can be very severe and there are indications that the mechanisms involved may be the same for all three drugs. The syndrome secondary to the use of these drugs has been described as a febrile state associated, among other events, with liver damage, and was initially called "Hypersensitivity Syndrome" [27].

Idiosyncrasy refers to the susceptibility of some individuals to the toxicity of a drug which, at conventional doses, is usually safe. Two general mechanisms have been proposed for idiosyncratic hepatotoxicity: metabolic idiosyncrasy and immuno-allergy. Metabolic idiosyncrasy can result from genetic or acquired alterations in drug metabolism, mitochondria, canalicular secretion or death receptor signaling. Immunoallergy refers to adverse reactions mediated by the immune system. These two mechanisms are probably interrelated[28].

Cases of idiosyncratic toxicity[29] account for 23% of 37% of drug-induced liver damage[30]. In addition, lipophilicity combined with dose, also known as the "rule of two" [31,32], is known to increase the risk of developing drug-induced liver damage, due to increased blood uptake in hepatocytes, forming greater quantities of reactive metabolites[29]. Metabolic mechanisms include oxidative stress, mitochondrial liability and inhibition of hepatobiliary transporters[29]. In the case of drug-induced and INH-induced liver damage, hepatocellular damage can result from the creation of covalent drug-protein adducts, leading to hapten formation and an immune response, and/or through direct mitochondrial damage by INH or its metabolites, leading to mitochondrial oxidative stress and impaired energy homeostasis[33]. If such mitochondrial deficiencies are already present, even non-toxic concentrations of INH can trigger marked hepatocellular damage due to the underlying impairment of complex I function [33].

Other examples of mitochondrial damage include: impaired beta-oxidation and mitochondrial respiration, membrane disruption and mtDNA damage, usually caused by tamoxifen, valproic acid, diclofenac and tacrine, respectively[29].

Clinically, drug-induced liver injury ranges from asymptomatic, acute or chronic hepatitis[34] to acute liver failure (ALF) or fulminant hepatic failure, defined as sudden, life-threatening liver dysfunction leading to coagulopathy and hepatic encephalopathy within 26 weeks of onset. Although severe drug-induced liver injury is rare clinically, drugs have become the leading overall cause of HAI in the United States and other Western countries[35]. In the United States, approximately 1600 to 2000 people a year develop HAI, with 30% of these patients receiving aggressive therapy including liver transplantation[36].

Acetaminophen (paracetamol) is the offending drug in 40%-50% of these cases, with a further 11%-12% of HAI cases being caused by herbal compounds and dietary supplements (HDS), equaling the frequency of HAI due to acute viral hepatitis and higher than that observed with all other individually identifiable causes[35, 37,38].

In fact, due to this significant morbidity and mortality, drug-induced liver injury continues to be a major reason for drugs being withdrawn from the market, with more recent examples including bromfenac and troglitazone[11]. Given the significant time and expense involved in bringing a new drug to market, it should come as no surprise that identifying potential toxicities early in the development process is paramount[39]. However, compounds cannot be guaranteed to be totally free of the potential to cause liver damage and injury in pre-clinical stages of development and, as such, tremendous strides have been made in regulatory science in order to identify drug-induced liver injury in clinical and post-approval settings[40,,42]. The creation of the Drug Induced Hepatotoxicity Assessment portion[43], the "Rule of Two" [31,32], FDA's Adverse Event Reporting System[44], Sentinel projects[45] and Hepatic Toxicity Knowledge Base[46] has empowered physicians to detect and predict drug-induced liver injury as early and successfully as possible. Working in parallel at the bedside, new hepatotoxins have been discovered, including dronedarone[47], ipilimumab[48, 49] and tolvaptan[50, 51] and our additional understanding of known hepatotoxins, including azithromycin[52], duloxetine[53], fluoroquinolones[54], statins[55], telithromycin[56], tyrosine kinase inhibitors[57] and others has been applied[58].

In addition, the identification of risk factors, predictors and biomarkers of injury[59- 67]and new mechanisms of injury[33, 68-72], together with refined causality assessment tools[73-75], and targeted hepatotoxicity treatment options[76-82], have come to define the current state of the art.

AEA are biotransformed into hydroxylated metabolites, which are stable and non-toxic by oxidation reactions mediated by cytochrome P450 isoenzymes. In this process, reactive intermediates are formed, areno-oxides, whose detoxification is carried out by epoxide hydrolases[83,84]. One mechanism suggested for the development of the idiosyncratic reaction associated with AEA is the accumulation of areno-oxide metabolites as a result of defects or deficiencies in the detoxification process by epoxide hydrolases[26].

Although there is clear evidence that the adverse reactions induced by AEA are mediated by an immune process, direct toxicity has also been suggested[18]. Areno-oxides are electrophilic, potentially toxic metabolites which, when not properly eliminated, can: (1) act as pro-hapten which bind to T-cells and initiate an immune response and/or (2) bind covalently (irreversibly) to biological macromolecules to directly or indirectly oxidize DNA, proteins and lipids, irreversibly altering cell function and leading to cell death[16,83]. The consequences of this interaction with cellular constituents vary depending on the different compounds formed and can result in necrosis, apoptosis, mutagenesis or teratogenesis[85, 86].

Drug-induced mitochondrial toxicity

The main way of eliminating reactive metabolites from the biotransformation of drugs is through conjugation reactions, mainly with glutathione. This tripeptide contains a thiol group capable of binding to electrophilic compounds directly or through reactions catalyzed by glutathione transferase, producing conjugates with mercapturic acid. Glutathione can also serve as a substrate in the elimination of peroxides resulting from the dismutation of the superoxide radical, a reaction catalyzed by different forms of glutathione peroxidase[87].

Experimental evidence indicates that mitochondria represent a preferential and critical target for the action of drugs and toxins[11, 88,8]9. Toxic effects on mitochondria can occur through direct and indirect mechanisms, including disruption of intracellular ion homeostasis, enzyme inhibition, damage to cell membranes and anoxia[90].

Numerous toxic agents are capable of interfering with the mechanisms responsible for maintaining cellular integrity. Many of these mechanisms depend on a constant supply of ATP to the cells. ATP is necessary for the activation of endogenous compounds through phosphorylation or adenylation, and can be incorporated into nucleic acids or used as a cofactor. It is necessary for muscle contraction, polymerization of the cytoskeleton, cell division, vesicular transport and maintenance of cell morphology. It is particularly important for the function of transporters such as Na /K^{++} -ATPase in the cytoplasmic membrane, Ca^{2+}-ATPase in the cytoplasmic membrane and endoplasmic reticulum and H^+ -ATPase in the lysosomal membrane. This set of transporters is essential for maintaining many cellular functions. The chemical energy needed to carry out this chemical, mechanical and osmotic work is provided by the hydrolysis of ATP to ADP or AMP. ADP is re-phosphorylated to ATP in the mitochondria by the enzyme FoF1-ATP synthetase, which works in conjunction with the reduction of oxygen to water, in a process known as oxidative phosphorylation[91].

F_0F_1-ATP synthase is the enzyme responsible for the mitochondrial synthesis of ATP, coupled to the electrochemical proton gradient, and catalyzes both the synthesis and hydrolysis of ATP. It is made up of a hydrophilic component (F_1), and one intrinsically associated with the membrane (F_o). The F_1 component contains the catalytic and regulatory sites, while Fo supposedly forms a proton channel through the inner membrane. The F_o and F_1 components are linked through the oligomycin sensitivity protein and the F6 component[91, 92]. Regarding the mechanisms involved in the catalytic sites of this enzyme, the experimental models proposed suggest that ATP synthesis and hydrolysis occur with the participation of three catalytic sites and that regulation occurs mainly through the interaction between F1 and an endogenous protein inhibitor[93].

During the transport of electrons transferred by oxidizable substrates to the respiratory chain, the mitochondria are able to generate an electrochemical gradient of protons in the inner membrane which, according to the chemiosmotic model proposed by Mitchell (1961), leads to the synthesis of ATP[94].

As well as supplying more than 95% of the energy used by the cell through oxidative phosphorylation, mitochondria play different roles in the regulation of various cellular processes, taking part in modulating the cell's redox state, osmotic regulation, pH control, cell signaling and, above all, maintaining calcium homeostasis. Due to this diversity of functions, mitochondria are target organelles for toxic agents and various damaging situations, and are involved in cell damage and death mechanisms[95].

Many agents are capable of interfering in the processes involved in oxidative phosphorylation, and they can be divided into uncouplers and inhibitors[96]. Uncouplers allow electron transport in the mitochondria, but prevent the phosphorylation of ADP to ATP by dissipating the electrochemical gradient, undoing the coupling between electron transport and ATP synthesis. 2,4-dinitrophenol and valinomycin are examples of this class of agents. Inhibitors act specifically on each complex of the respiratory chain: rotenone blocks the transport of electrons from NADH to ubiquinone; antimycin A blocks the transfer of electrons from ubiquinone to cytochrome c and cyanide blocks the reduction of oxygen by cytochrome aa_3. Agents such as fluoracetate, which inhibit the Krebs cycle with a consequent decrease in the generation of reduced cofactors, also decrease oxidative phosphorylation. Atractyloside, a toxic glycoside of plant origin, inhibits the enzyme adenine nucleotide translocase, preventing cytosolic ADP from being transported into the mitochondria to be reconverted into ATP, and the ATP produced inside the mitochondria from being transported into the cytosol. Finally, there are F_oF_1-ATPase inhibitors, such as oligomycin, which binds to the F_o portion of the enzyme in a mitochondrial membrane-dependent bond, inhibiting ATP synthesis[91].

There is evidence that some drugs exert pharmacological and/or toxicological effects by interacting with the mechanisms involved in energy production by mitochondria. This is the case with some psychoactive compounds, such as reserpine, butyrophenones, phenothiazines, tricyclic antidepressants, valproate and benzodiazepines. Imipramine and its analogues, widely used tricyclic antidepressants, have a marked effect on mitochondrial oxidative phosphorylation in various tissues, as well as high solubility in the mitochondrial membrane[97,98].

Neuroleptics, drugs prescribed to millions of patients, have their clinical use limited by their extrapyramidal side effects, similar to the neurotoxin 1-methyl-4- phenyl-1,2,3,6-tetrahydropyridine, which produces parkinsonism, apparently by inhibiting NADH:ubiquinone oxidoreductase (complex I) of the electron transport chain. Similarly, chlorpromazine and thiothixin also inhibit complex I *in* brain mitochondria *in vitro*. Clonazine, an atypical antipsychotic, has few extrapyramidal effects, but inhibits complex I at high concentrations[99].

Benzodiazepines, which are widely used as muscle relaxants, anticonvulsants, sedative hypnotics and anxiolytics, exert their effect by binding specifically to CNS receptors: central benzodiazepine receptors, coupled to GABA and chloride channels[100]. In addition, benzodiazepines bind to other receptors

They are localized in the mitochondria and are therefore called mitochondrial benzodiazepine receptors[101]. Mitochondrial benzodiazepine receptors appear to be involved in the modulation of various physiological functions, such as cell growth and differentiation, calcium homeostasis[102] and lipid metabolism, including the secretion of steroid hormones[103]. Benzodiazepines also affect the respiratory control of mitochondria[104].

Oxidative Stress

During various pathological/toxicological processes, excessive production of reactive oxygen species can cause lipoperoxidation of mitochondrial membrane systems and/or an increase in permeability known as mitochondrial membrane permeability transition (MMPT). This phenomenon is dependent on the opening of a non-selective pore with the participation of calcium ions and an inducing agent such as: pro-oxidizing substances, Pi, or uncouplers of oxidative phosphorylation. This apparent increase in permeability may be a key event in the course of a series of toxic and pathological processes and apoptosis. Thus, agents that induce TPMM as well as lipoperoxidation of the mitochondrial membrane may be of toxicological interest[105].

Lipoperoxidation begins with the action of any species capable of subtracting a hydrogen from the polyunsaturated fatty acids in membranes. In this way, a peroxyl radical is formed. This radical can attack an adjacent fatty acid and thus propagate the reaction (lipid peroxidation). In this way, a series of reactions is established and peroxides accumulate in the membrane. Peroxidized lipids destabilize the membrane and cause ions to leak out. Peroxyl radicals can attack not only lipids, but also membrane proteins, damaging enzymes, receptors and signal transduction systems, as well as oxidizing cholesterol[105].

The most sensitive proteins are those with thiol groups in their structure. Modification of the structure of these proteins by oxidative stress is usually accompanied by a weakening of various cellular functions, such as inhibition of phosphoinositide metabolism, disruption of intracellular calcium homeostasis and the cell's normal cytoskeleton. This last effect may be responsible for the formation of vesicles in the plasma membrane, observed in cells exposed to cytotoxic concentrations of pro-oxidants[106].

The electron transport chain has been recognized as the main intracellular source of reactive oxygen species (ROS). In the presence of various drugs or toxins, such as electron transport chain inhibitors, oxidative phosphorylation uncouplers, quinonoid compounds and metals, the generation of free oxygen radicals by mitochondria can be substantially increased[106]. The superoxide anion radical (O_2^- ·) appears to be the main product of incomplete oxygen reduction under physiological and pathological conditions. Under the action of superoxide dismutase, the superoxide radical is transformed into hydrogen peroxide (H_2O_2), the reduction of which can lead to the hydroxyl radical (OII*). While part of the superoxide and hydrogen peroxide can diffuse out of the mitochondria and damage cellular components far from their site of formation, hydroxyl, due to its high reactivity and consequent very short half-life, has no diffusion capacity. Thus, the effects of ROS may be greater in the inner mitochondrial membrane, whose main component of the phospholipid bilayer is cardiolipin, a derivative of diphosphatidyl glycerol, which has a high ratio of unsaturated to saturated fatty acids. Cardiolipin plays an important role in controlling membrane permeability, as well as establishing the electrochemical proton gradient. It is also a regulator of state 3 respiration and can modulate the secondary structure of proteins in the inner mitochondrial membrane, such as substrate transporters,

NADI dehydrogenase, cytochrome bc1, cytochrome c oxidase and ATP synthase[107]. In addition, the inner mitochondrial membrane has enzymes containing iron and copper, which can catalyze the reaction of superoxide and I2O2 [108].

The mitochondria have a complex antioxidant defense system, consisting of the enzymes superoxide dismutase (SOD), glutathione peroxidase, glutathione reductase and glutathione transferase, as well as non-enzymatic oxidants such as reduced glutathione (GSH), NADPI, vitamin C and vitamin E[109]. Under conditions of excess ROS production in the mitochondria, their defense system may be insufficient to neutralize these radicals, leading to a situation known as oxidative stress[110].

The generation of reactive oxygen species by the mitochondria is a continuous and physiologically normal process under aerobic conditions, and around 1-2% of the oxygen reduced by the mitochondria is converted to superoxide[111].

The most important defense against oxidative damage induced by reactive oxygen species is the maintenance of glutathione (GSH) homeostasis. Reduced glutathione serves as a substrate for the action of: (1) glutathione peroxidase, in the removal of hydrogen peroxide produced by the action of superoxide dismutase on the superoxide radical; (2) glutathione transferase in the formation of mercapturic acid and the elimination of xenobiotics; as well as acting as a free radical scavenger. It also acts as an intracellular regulator of disulfide thiols in glycolytic enzymes and ATPase-Ca++ 112. The action of glutathione peroxidase leads to the production of glutathione disulfide (GSSG) or oxidized glutathione. In its oxidized form, glutathione is toxic to the cell due to the formation of cysteinyl derivatives, especially in the presence of transition metals[113,114].

The reactions dependent on reduced glutathione are of fundamental importance for protecting the cell against oxidative stress, as they keep the cell in a reduced environment under normal physiological conditions. The breakdown of thiol homeostasis in cells treated with pro-oxidants causes a weakening of the calcium translocation system, stimulation of calcium channels, and inhibition of calcium sequestration by the endoplasmic reticulum and mitochondria. This results in the cell's inability to maintain intracellular calcium concentration at physiological levels. The breakdown of intracellular calcium homeostasis is associated with the progression of cell damage[115].

Intracellular calcium homeostasis

Calcium can be transported from the cytosol to the mitochondrial matrix using the energy of the electrochemical proton gradient in the mitochondria's inner membrane. Influx occurs in response to the negative potential inside the membrane, while efflux occurs through exchange with H^+ from the outside, or with sodium from the cytosol. Among other factors, the cytosolic concentration of calcium is the result of the balance between efflux and influx of the cation into the mitochondria. Although calcium plays an important regulatory role, activating mitochondrial dehydrogenases, its presence in non-physiological concentrations is responsible for compromising mitochondrial energy function[115].

Calcium is a biologically very active ion and is involved in the regulation of various cellular processes; an increase in cytosolic calcium levels causes the activation of various calcium-dependent enzyme systems, including phospholipases, dehydrogenases, proteases and endonucleases, and this increase can be critical in a variety of pathophysiological and toxicological processes. The mitochondrial calcium cycle, determined by the influx and efflux of the ion, could protect the cell from large cytosolic variations that occur in response to various situations, such as ischemia-reperfusion, the toxic action of heavy metals and other adverse situations [116]. It is also believed that the formation of reactive oxygen species, the oxidation of thiol groups in mitochondrial membrane proteins and a decrease in the cell's reducing power are events involved in the cell damage caused by an increase in the cytosolic concentration of calcium[117].

The mitochondria have the ability to rapidly sequester large amounts of calcium, thus limiting its harmful effects on the cell. This influx occurs through a specific transporter that mainly uses the energy of the electrochemical proton gradient. Several studies have shown that mitochondria cannot sequester calcium in the absence of membrane potential[118].

Calcium in high concentrations, or in the presence of inorganic phosphate, pro-oxidants and uncouplers, can cause a rapid change in the permeability of the inner mitochondrial membrane, associated with membrane depolarization, uncoupling of oxidative phosphorylation, loss of metabolic intermediates, release of intramitochondrial ions and large-scale mitochondrial swelling resulting from loss of selectivity of the inner mitochondrial membrane[119]. This event, known as mitochondrial membrane permeability transition (MMPT), is calcium-dependent and is associated with the formation of disulfide bridges in mitochondrial membrane proteins[120], and can be reversed by EGTA[111]. In addition, the oxidation of pyridine nucleotides and the generation of reactive oxygen species can induce PMS[119]. Previous studies have shown that during the oxidation of pyridine nucleotides, calcium is released from the mitochondria. The reduction of these nucleotides by oxidizable substrates reverses this situation, causing an influx of calcium into the mitochondria[96,121] .

Since TPMM and the subsequent events (mitochondrial swelling, dissipation of membrane potential, breakdown of calcium homeostasis and cellular energy failure) are involved in the processes of cell damage and death, the study of drugs that alter these events is important for: (1) establishing their toxicological potential and (2) delineating the biochemical mechanisms involved.

Relevance of the Study and Future Prospects

Little is known about non-immune forms of drug-induced idiosyncratic hepatotoxicity[122]. Chemically reactive metabolites have been proposed as responsible for many types of drug-induced hepatotoxicity, but evidence on the role of these metabolites in such events is difficult to obtain due to the lack of appropriate *in vitro* and *in vivo* models. Furthermore, the mechanisms by which these metabolites initiate and propagate cell damage are still poorly understood[7]. The direct toxicity of reactive metabolites may involve mitochondrial dysfunction, one of the most important mechanisms of drug-induced liver damage. Mitochondria are the point of convergence of the different signals that culminate in hepatocyte death, regardless of the type of cell death induced: apoptosis, necrosis or autophagy[122]. The effects of AEA on mitochondrial function have not yet been clarified. Knowledge of the mechanisms involved in the idiosyncratic hepatotoxicity associated with the use of AEA can contribute to: (1) the development of adjuvant liver protection therapies and (2) the prevention of liver damage by establishing predisposing factors and the profile of susceptible individuals.

Therefore, in order to expand our knowledge, we saw the importance of evaluating the potential of carbamazepine, phenytoin and phenobarbital to interfere *in* cellular bioenergetic processes, by investigating the *in vitro* effects of the unchanged drugs or their reactive metabolites (areno-oxides) on mitochondria isolated from rat liver.

METHODS

Experimental Model

All the studies were carried out *in vitro*. Both the direct effect of the drugs and their respective metabolites (areno-oxides) generated *in vitro* by incubating each drug with the rat liver microsomal system were evaluated.

Studies carried out:

A. Studies related to mitochondrial respiration

- Oxygen consumption in state 3 (activated) of respiration
- Oxygen consumption in state 4 (non-activated) of respiration
- Determination of the Respiratory Control Ratio (RCR)

B. Studies related to Mitochondrial Membrane Permeability Transition

- Mitochondrial osmotic swelling
- Mitochondrial membrane potential
- Calcium uptake and release

C. Studies related to oxidative stress

- Determination of malondialdehyde (MDA) - lipoperoxidation

- Determination of sulfhydryl protein
- Determination of carbonylated proteins
- Mitochondrial redox state: GSH/GSSG ratio
- Determination of cardiolipin

Isolation of Mitochondria from Rat Liver

The animals were sacrificed by cervical dislocation and the liver (10-15 grams) of each animal was immediately removed and minced into 50 ml of a medium containing 250 mM sucrose, 1 mM EGTA and 10 mM Hepes-KOH, pH 7.4 and homogenized in a Potter-Elvehjem homogenizer (3 cycles of 15 seconds with one-minute intervals). The mitochondria were isolated according to the procedure described by Pedersen et al. (1978), with some modifications. The homogenate was centrifuged at 770 x g for 5 minutes, and the resulting supernatant was centrifuged at 9,800 x g for 10 minutes. The precipitate was returned to 10 ml of a medium containing 250 mM sucrose, 0.3 mM EGTA and 10 mM Hepes-KOH, pH 7.4 and centrifuged at 4,500 x g for 15 minutes. The mitochondrial precipitate was suspended in 1 ml of a medium containing 250 mM sucrose and 10 mM Hepes-KOH, pH 7.4 at a concentration of 20 mg mitochondrial protein/ml. All procedures were carried out at 4°C and the mitochondrial solution was used within a maximum of 3 hours after isolation. The solutions were prepared with bi-distilled and deionized water. Each experiment was repeated using 3 to 6 different mitochondrial preparations.

Mitochondrial Protein Determination

Protein was determined according to the method described by Bradford (1976), using bovine serum albumin (BSA) as a standard. To 25 µl of the mitochondrial suspension was added 10 ml of the coloring reagent composed of Coomassie 250 R 0.01% (w/v), methanol 8.5% (v/v) and phosphoric acid 85% (v/v). After stirring and standing for 5 minutes, the absorbance was determined at 595 nm against the color reagent.

Preparation of liver microsomes

The animals were pre-treated with phenobarbital (10 mg/kg, intraperitoneally, 3 days) to induce the cytochrome P-450 system. The animals then remained without food for 24 hours and were sacrificed by cervical dislocation. The livers were removed, washed in 0.9% NaCl (immersed in an ice bath) and cut into small pieces. Portions of 5 g of liver were added to 15 mL of 150 mM KCl (immersed in an ice bath) and homogenized in Potter-Elvehjem (3 times for 15 seconds, 1 minute apart). The homogenate thus obtained was centrifuged at 9,000 x *g* for 10 min at 4°C. The resulting supernatant (fraction S9) was centrifuged at 100,000 x *g* for 60 min at 4°C. The precipitate thus obtained was returned to 10 mL of 150 mM KCl (ice-cold), centrifuged at 100,000 x *g* at 4°C for 30 min and again returned to 10 mL of 150 mM KCl, immersed in an ice bath (microsomal fraction) ([123]).

In vitro toxicity tests induced by drugs and metabolites

The *in vitro* toxicity test induced by areno-oxides in human lymphocytes, previously described by Spielberg et al. (1981), was modified and adapted for the assessment of mitochondrial liver toxicity. The concentrations of the drugs (0.025 mM - 1 mM) used in the tests were also chosen on the basis of the study mentioned above. The incubation medium was composed of 210 mM mannitol, 70 mM sucrose, 10 mM Hepes-Na, 1 mM EGTA, 0.01% BSA, 2.4 mM glucose-6-phosphate, 0.6 mM NADP and 2 U glucose-6-phosphate dehydrogenases. The tests were carried out under three different experimental conditions: (A) control: mitochondrial protein (5mg/mL); (B) unchanged drug: mitochondrial protein (5 mg/mL) together with different concentrations (0.025 mM - 1mM) of each drug; (C) bioactivated drug: mitochondrial protein (5 mg/mL) together with microsomal protein (Img/mL) and different concentrations (0.025 mM - 1 mM) of each drug. The volume of the drug solutions never exceeded 20 μL to ensure that the vehicle used (DMSO) did not interfere with the assays. After the end of the incubation, the mitochondrial suspensions were centrifuged at 10,000g for 10 minutes and resumed in 250 mM sucrose and 10mM Hepes-Na, pH 7.4. The final concentration was adjusted to 20 mg of mitochondrial protein/ml, except for the mitochondria used to determine the mitochondrial protein.

MDA, which was then replenished with 150 mM KCl and 5 mM Tris-HCl, pH 7.4 and adjusted to a final concentration of 1 mg of mitochondrial protein/ml.

Studies related to mitochondrial respiration

- ***Determination of Oxygen Consumption (states 3 and 4) and RCR***

Oxygen consumption was analyzed polarographically at 30°C on an oximeter equipped with a Clark electrode (Gilson Medical Electronics, USA).

The respiratory substrates 5 mM potassium succinate + 1 μg/ml rotenone or 5 mM potassium glutamate + 5mM potassium malate were incubated in a respiration medium containing: 125 mM sucrose, 65 mM KCl, 10 mM potassium phosphate, 0.5 mM EGTA and 10 mM Hepes-KOH, pH 7.4 at 30°C, in order to obtain a final volume of 1.5 ml. 1 mg of mitochondrial protein was used in each assay and respiration was initiated by the addition of 0.5 μmol of ADP. The Respiratory Control Ratio (RCR), as well as O_2 consumption in states 3 (activated) and 4 of respiration (non-activated) were determined from the polarographic tracing, according to the method described by Estrabook (1967)[124].

Studies related to Mitochondrial Membrane Permeability Transition

♦ ***Mitochondrial Osmotic Swelling***

The mitochondria (0.4 mg of protein) were incubated in 1.5 ml of a medium containing: 125 mM sucrose, 65 mM KCl, 2 mM potassium succinate, 5 μM rotenone and 10 mM Hepes-KOH, pH 7.4, at 30OC and the changes in absorbance were determined at 540 nm. Swelling was initiated by the addition of 10 μM of CaCl2 and after 2 minutes, 1.5 mM of potassium phosphate or 500 μM of the drugs were added.

♦ ***Mitochondrial Membrane Potential***

The electrical potential of the inner mitochondrial membrane was assessed by monitoring the mitochondrial uptake of rhodamine 123 using a fluorescence spectrometer (F-2500, Hitachi) operating at 535 nm (emission) and 505 nm (excitation). 1 mg of mitochondrial protein was used and the incubation medium was composed as follows: KCl 160 mM, potassium phosphate 8.5 mM, HEPES-KOH 10 mM, pH 7.4, rotenone 5 μM and rhodamine (123) 5 μM. 10 mM succinate was used as the respiratory substrate. The reaction was initiated by the addition of 0.4 μmol ADP and the assay was carried out at 30°C[125].

♦ ***Determination of Mitochondrial Calcium Release***

The kinetics of calcium release by liver mitochondria was determined using Arsenazo III at 675-685 nm (Scarpa, 1979). The incubation medium (final volume of 1 mL) was composed of 125 mM sucrose, 65 mM KCl, 5 μM rotenone, 5 mM potassium succinate, 25 μM arsenazo III, and 10 mM Hepes-KOH, pH 7.4, at 30OC, in the absence or presence of 20 μM $CaCl_2$.

♦ **Mitochondrial calcium uptake/release**

The uptake/release of calcium by the mitochondria (1 mg of protein) was monitored as described above for the calcium release assays. The incubation medium was composed of 125 mM sucrose, 65 mM KCl, 5 μM rotenone, 25 μM arsenazo III, 20 μM $CaCl_2$, and 10 mM Hepes-KOH, pH 7.4, at 30OC. Calcium uptake was initiated by the addition of 5 mM potassium succinate.

Studies related to Oxidative Stress

♦ ***Determination of MDA (lipoperoxidation)***

Freshly isolated mitochondria (0.5 mg) were incubated in an Erlenmeyer flask under agitation (100 cycles/minute) for 15 minutes at 30°C in a medium containing 125 mM sucrose, 65 mM KCl, 5mM glutamate+ 5mM malate, 1μg rotenone, 20μM Fe++ 100 μM ADP and 10 mM Hepes-KOH, pH 7.4 (final volume 1 ml). The incubation conditions were as follows: (1) in the presence of 500 μM of carbamazepine, phenytoin or phenobarbital; (2) in the presence of the vehicle (DMSO) used to solubilize the drug (negative control); (3) in the presence of 0.5 mM of t-butylhydroperoxide (positive control). The reaction was completed by adding 2 ml of a solution of 0.35% thiobarbituric acid in 0.25 mM HCl and 15% trichloroacetic acid. The resulting mixture was left to stand for 12 hours in the dark and the resulting staining was determined at 533 nm. The amount of MDA was calculated using the molar extinction coefficient of 1.49 x 105 M-1 126.

- ***Determination of Protein Sulfhydryl (P-SH)***

After 15 minutes of incubation, the mitochondria were treated with perchloric acid (final concentration 7%) to precipitate the proteins, and centrifuged at 4,500 x g for 5 minutes. The precipitate was suspended with 100 µl of perchloric acid, supplemented with 1 ml of water and centrifuged at 4,500 x g for 5 minutes. The final precipitate was recovered with 0.2 ml of 10% Triton X-100 and 0.8 ml of water. A 0.2 ml aliquot of 500 mM potassium phosphate, pH 7.6 was added to 0.8 ml of the suspension. The amount of sulfhydryl groups was determined by the difference in absorbance at 412 nm before and 5 minutes after the addition of DTNB (final concentration 0.2 M). A molar extinction coefficient of 13,600 M-1 was used.

- ***Determination of Carbonylated Proteins (CP)***

The mitochondrial suspension (9 parts) was treated with 10% streptomycin sulfate in HEPES, pH 7.2 (1 part), and after 15 minutes centrifuged at 10,000 x g for 5 minutes. To 300 µl of the supernatant was added 300 µl of 0.2% 2,4-dinitro-phenylhydrazine in 2M HCl. After 1 hour of incubation at 25°C, 50 µl of 50% TCA were added and the mixture centrifuged at 10,000 x g for 5 minutes. The sediment was washed three times with 1.0 ml of a 1/1 (v/v) ethanol/ethyl acetate mixture and dissolved in 2.0 ml of 6M guanidine in 20 mM sodium phosphate buffer, pH 6.5. The absorbance was determined at 365 nm against a reference under the same conditions, replacing the dinitro-phenylhydrazine solution with an equal volume of 2 M HCl solution. The molar extinction coefficient of 22,000 M^{-1} x cm^{-1} [127] was used to determine the concentration.

- *Determination of Reduced Glutathione (GSH) and Oxidized Glutathione (GSSG)*

After the incubation period, the solution was centrifuged at 10,000 x g for 10 minutes. The mitochondrial precipitate was treated with 500µl of 6% $HClO_4$ and centrifuged at 10,000 x g for 10 minutes. For GSH determination, 50 µl of the supernatant was added to a reaction medium composed of 0.1 M potassium phosphate buffer, pH 7.2, 1 mM EDTA and 0.3 mM NADPH. After 5 minutes at 30°C, the reaction was started with 0.5 U of glutathione reductase and the absorbance was determined at 412 nm for 5 minutes. For the determination of GSSG, 200 µl of the supernatant was added to 100 µg of sodium carbonate and 4 µl of 2- vinylpyridine. After resting for 1 hour in the dark, the mixture was centrifuged at 3,000 x g for 5 minutes and 100 µl of the supernatant was submitted to the procedure described above for the GSH assay [128]. The concentrations of GSH and GSSG were calculated from calibration curves obtained under the same experimental conditions.

♦ *Determination of Cardiolipin*

After incubation, the mitochondria were labeled with N-nonyl-acridine orange (NAO) at a concentration of 100 nmol/mg of protein and after 2 minutes the mitochondria were centrifuged at 30,000 x g for 5 minutes. In the case of mitochondria that had undergone the bioactivation process, they were labeled directly with NAO and then centrifuged at 30,000 x g for 5 minutes. In both situations, the absorbance of the supernatant was determined at 495 nm [129].

RESULTS

Effects on mitochondrial respiration

All the bioactivated drugs were able to: increase oxygen consumption in state 4 (Fig. 1); decrease oxygen consumption in state 3 (Fig. 2) and consequently decrease RCR (Fig. 3). The RCR (Respiratory Control Ratio) represents the ratio between the

oxygen consumed after the addition of ADP (state 3) and the oxygen consumed in basal respiration (state 4, not activated by ADP).

State 4 of respiration was not affected by any of the unchanged drugs, however, at high concentrations (from 200 μM; CI50 of approximately 750 μM), unchanged phenobarbital promoted inhibition of state 3 respiration (Fig.2), as well as a decrease in RCR (Fig.3).

In the case of phenytoin, in its unchanged form it did not affect mitochondrial function, but after bioactivation it became extremely active, and at a concentration of 50 μM it already caused a significant increase in state 4 of respiration ($p<0.01$). The maximum uncoupling effect was obtained at a concentration of 100 μM and an inhibitory effect was observed from this concentration onwards. The CI_{50} (concentration causing 50% inhibition) was 75 μM (Fig. 1). In relation to state 3, the effects were milder, with a statistically significant inhibitory effect ($p<0.001$) only being obtained at a concentration of 200 μM, which remained relatively constant at higher concentrations (Fig. 2). The RCR began to decrease at a concentration of 25 μM ($p<0.05$), and from 200 μM the mitochondria were completely uncoupled, an event characterized by RCR=1 (Fig. 3). A similar behavior was obtained in the tests with carbamazepine. In its unchanged form, carbamazepine had no effect on mitochondrial function, but after bioactivation, it also had an uncoupling effect, but only at higher concentrations and with less intensity when compared to phenytoin and phenobarbital. State 4 of respiration only began to be altered from a concentration of 100 μM ($p<0.05$) and the maximum uncoupling effect was not reached at the concentrations used (Fig. 1). With regard to state 3, there was a marked difference compared to the other two drugs, as an initial increase in oxygen consumption was observed at concentrations of 50-100 μM (Fig. 2). This oxygen consumption remained higher compared to the control and compensated for the uncoupling effect in such a way that the RCR was only significantly altered from 500 μM onwards, without the maximum theoretical inhibition (RCR=1) being reached (Fig. 3).

Phenobarbital, which in its unchanged form already had a reasonable inhibitory effect, when subjected to the bioactivation process also exerted an uncoupling effect (increased basal oxygen consumption). State 4 was altered from 50 μM ($p<0.01$) and reached its maximum peak at 500 μM, with a maximum inhibitory effect already observed at 1000 μM (Fig. 1). Its inhibitory effect on state 3 (Fig. 2) was apparently abolished by the increase in state 4. However, when analyzing the RCR, the relationship between these two stages of respiration, it can be seen that this apparent compensation did not occur, as the RCR was drastically affected, and at a concentration of 100 μM there was already about a 95% reduction in its value (Fig. 3).

The data shown in Figs. 1, 2 and 3 were obtained using glutamate and malate as respiratory substrates. In the studies with succinate or ascorbate/TMPD as respiratory substrates (data not shown), the pattern of behavior for the 3 drugs analyzed was similar to those obtained with glutamate/malate, which demonstrates that the bioactivated drugs exert inhibitory effects in a non-specific way on the three sites of the respiratory chain.

Fig. 4 shows the inhibition of state 3 respiration by different concentrations of phenobarbital (500 and 1000 μM), as well as the amount of oxygen consumed by the mitochondria. While in the control trials 150 n atoms of O/mg protein/min were consumed, in the trials with 500 μM phenobarbital this value fell to 103 n atoms of O/mg protein/min and in the trials with 1000 μM the consumption was only 50 n atoms of O/mg protein/min. Thus, the estimated value for CI_{50} was approximately 750 μM. Similar CI_{50} values were also obtained for respiration supported by succinate, site 2 substrate, and by ascorbate/TMPD, site 3 substrate (data not shown).

Fig. 5(A) shows the influence of unchanged phenobarbital on glutamate/malate oxidation, stimulated by ADP (state 3 of respiration) or by the CCCP uncoupler. For comparison, the effects of the oxidative phosphorylation inhibitors are shown in Fig. 5(B), which shows that the inhibition pattern of the drug was similar to those caused by site 1 (rotenone, Rot), site 2 (antimycin A, Ant A) and site 3 (KCN) respiratory chain inhibitors. The effect was observed in both ADP- and CCCP-stimulated respiration. Furthermore, in contrast to what was observed for oligomycin (F_0F_1-ATPase inhibitor) and atractyloside (ADP/ATP transporter inhibitor), the inhibition of ADP-stimulated respiration was not altered by the uncoupler CCCP, when in the presence of the drug. A similar pattern of inhibition was also observed when succinate/rotenone or ascorbate/TMPD were used as respiratory substrates (Fig. 6).

Effects on ATP synthesis

Phenobarbital was the only unchanged drug that inhibited ATP synthesis, which would be expected considering its effect on mitochondrial respiration. The CI_{50} was 750 μM. The bioactivation of phenobarbital intensified its effect on ATP synthesis, and its CI50 was 750 μM.

CI_{50} was reduced to around 200 μM and its maximum inhibitory activity, which was 30%, increased to 55%. Phenytoin proved to be highly inhibitory, with an IC_{50} of approximately 100 μM and a onset of activity at a low concentration (50 μM). Carbamazepine had the least effect on ATP synthesis compared to the other bioactivated drugs, and its IC_{50} value was 1000 μM, the highest of the three (Fig. 7).

Inducing Oxidative Stress

None of the three unchanged drugs showed any pro-oxidant or antioxidant activity in relation to the oxidative stress indicators studied (Table 2). For comparison, the results obtained with t-butyl hydroperoxide (positive control) as well as in the absence of the drugs (negative control) are also shown in Table 2: it can be seen that the values obtained in the presence of the unchanged drugs are very close to those obtained in the negative control. Complementing these findings, the inclusion of superoxide dismutase and catalase during the mitochondrial respiration assay did not result in any protective effect on state 3 inhibition induced by phenobarbital, eliminating a possible involvement of reactive oxygen species in this process (data not shown).

After the bioactivation process, the three drugs promoted intense lipoperoxidation, altering all the oxidative stress indicators evaluated (malondialdehyde, glutathione, carbonylated protein and sulfhydryl protein). Bioactivated phenytoin promoted intense lipoperoxidation, followed by bioactivated phenobarbital and carbamazepine, which can be seen in the malondialdehyde (MDA) values found (Fig. 8). Cardiolipin, the main lipid fraction of the inner mitochondrial membrane, was also particularly oxidized by bioactivated phenytoin, with the effect starting as early as 50μM. Bioactivated carbamazepine had the least intense effect on cardiolipin (only from 200μM) and phenobarbital had an intermediate effect (Fig. 9). In line with these findings, the oxidation of mitochondrial proteins occurred in a similar way, i.e. among the 3 bioactivated drugs, phenytoin caused the most intense effect, and carbamazepine caused the least intense effect. The two tests showing these effects, oxidation of sulfhydryl groups and formation of carbonyl groups, are shown in Figures 10 and 11 respectively.

The mitochondrial redox state was also affected by the bioactivated drugs, which can be seen by the change in the GSH/GSSG ratio, i.e. there was a decrease in the levels of the reduced form of glutathione, accompanied by an increase in the levels of oxidized glutathione. Bioactivated phenytoin had the most intense effect at the lowest concentration (50µM) (Figs. 12 and 13).

Effects related to Mitochondrial Membrane Permeability Transition (MMPT)

The unchanged drugs had no effect on the mitochondria's ability to release or capture calcium (Fig. 14A); establish membrane potential (Figs. 15A and 15B); and neither induced (data not shown) nor inhibited mitochondrial swelling (Fig. 16A). As unchanged phenobarbital has an inhibitory effect on state 3 respiration, only a small drop in membrane potential was observed after the addition of ADP (Fig. 15B).

On the other hand, the intense lipoperoxidation promoted by the bioactivated drugs affected the mitochondria's ability to capture/release calcium (Fig.14B), to form and maintain membrane potential (Figs. 15C, 15D and 15E), as well as to swell (Fig. 16B), phenomena that are related to and totally dependent on the integrity of the mitochondria's membrane systems.

In relation to calcium transport, at a concentration of 200µM bioactivated phenytoin not only inhibited total calcium uptake by around 50%, but also promoted its rapid release. The same effect was observed with bioactivated phenobarbital, but at higher concentrations (from 500 µM). Carbamazepine (200 µM) was unable to significantly alter calcium uptake/release (Fig. 14B).

In the case of bioactivated phenytoin, at a concentration of 50µM, the membrane potential was formed, which fell in the presence of ADP as a result of the phosphorylation of ADP to ATP, returned to its previous levels, but was not maintained as expected, falling apart spontaneously (Fig. 15C). At a concentration of 200 µM, the potential was formed, but it was not maintained and there was no response to the addition of ADP. The same effect was observed with 500µM of bioactivated phenobarbital (Fig. 15B). At a concentration of 500µM bioactivated phenytoin completely inhibited the formation of the membrane potential (Fig. 15D). Bioactivated carbamazepine, on the other hand, was less effective in altering the membrane potential, since at a high concentration (500µM) the potential was still formed, there was a response to ADP (phosphorylation to ATP) and the potential was recomposed, which remained stable (Fig. 15E).

The effects of the bioactivated drugs on calcium uptake and release were directly reflected in mitochondrial swelling, as this event did not occur even in the presence of the inducer Pi (Fig.16B). One of the possible causes of this finding could be the inability of mitochondria to maintain intracellular calcium, which is essential for mitochondrial swelling to occur.

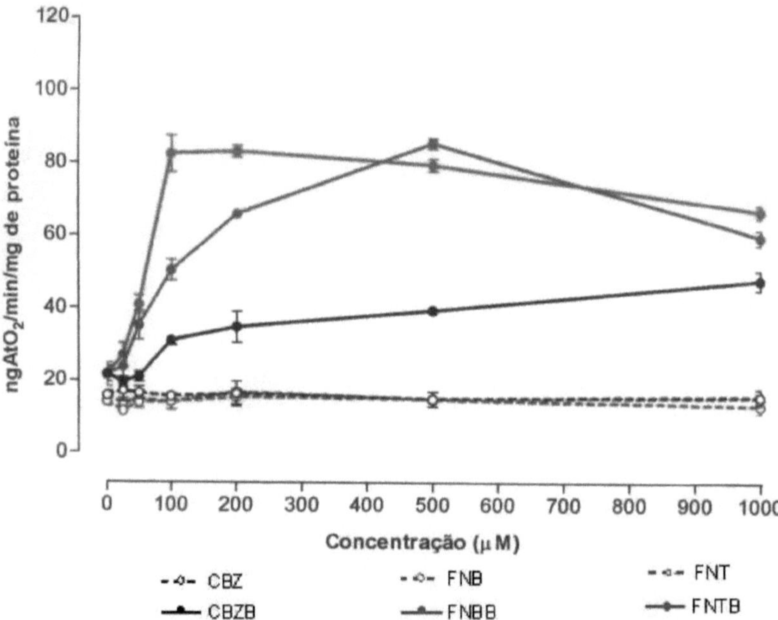

FIGURA 1. Effects of unchanged and bioactivated drugs (carbamazepine, phenobarbital and phenytoin) on state 4 of mitochondrial respiration (n=6; glutamate+ malate). The test conditions are described in Materials and Methods. CBZ = unchanged carbamazepine; CBZB = bioactivated carbamazepine; FNB = unchanged phenobarbital; FNBB = bioactivated phenobarbital; FNT = phenytoin; FNTB = bioactivated phenytoin.

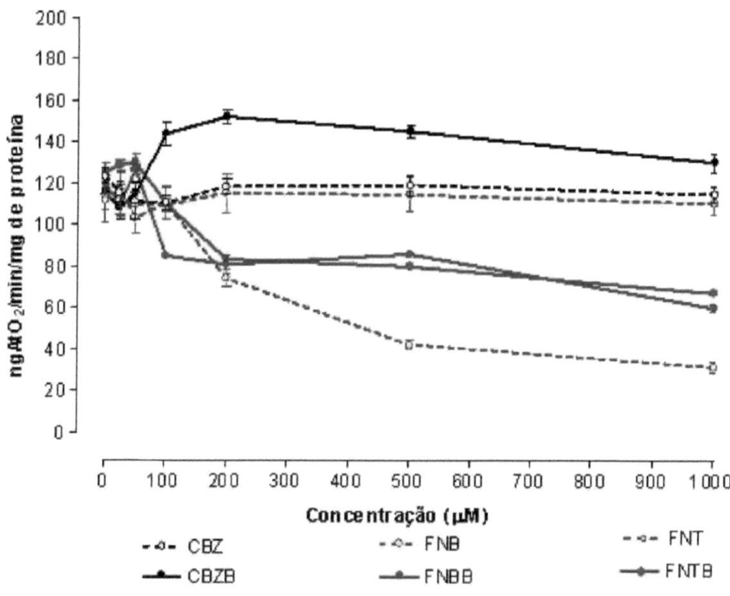

FIGURA 2. Effects of unchanged and bioactivated drugs (carbamazepine, phenobarbital and phenytoin) on state 3 of mitochondrial respiration (n=6; glutamate+ malate). The test conditions are described in Materials and Methods. CBZ = unchanged carbamazepine; CBZB = bioactivated carbamazepine; FNB = unchanged phenobarbital; FNBB = bioactivated phenobarbital; FNT = phenytoin; FNTB = bioactivated phenytoin.

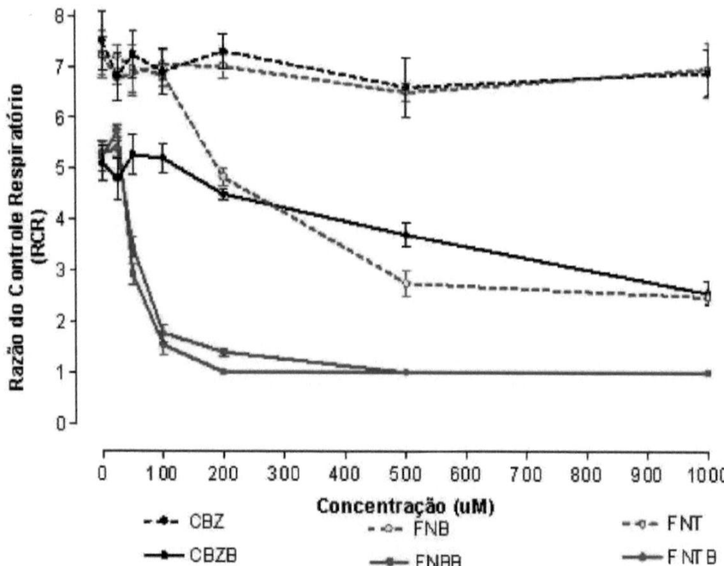

FIGURA 3. Effects of unchanged and bioactivated drugs (carbamazepine, phenobarbital and phenytoin) on the mitochondrial Respiratory Control Ratio (RCR) (n=6; glutamate+ malate). The assay conditions are described in Materials and Methods. CBZ = carbamazepine unchanged; CBZB= carbamazepine bioactivated; FNB= phenobarbital unchanged; FNBB = phenobarbital bioactivated; FNT = phenytoin; FNTB = phenytoin bioactivated.

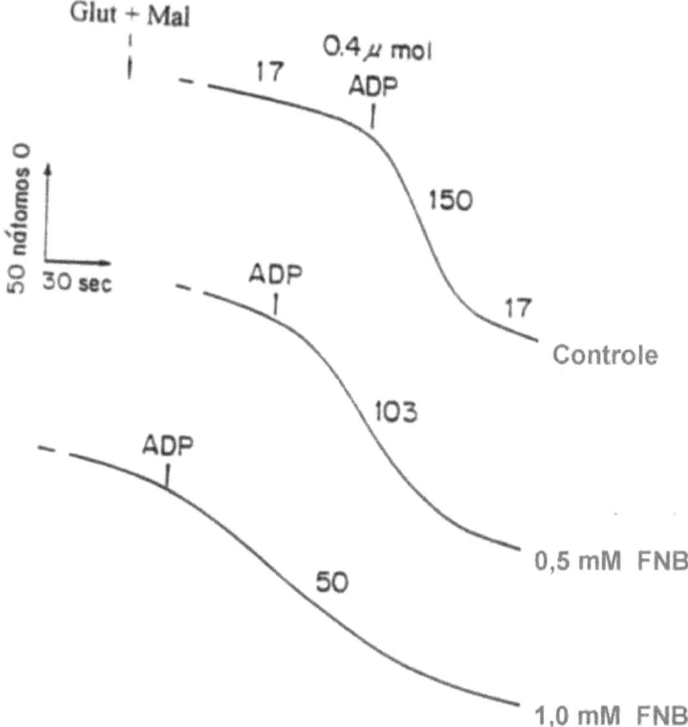

FIGURE 4 - Effect of unchanged phenobarbital (FNB) on the oxidation of malate+ glutamate by rat liver mitochondria. The values were expressed as number of O atoms/mg protein/min. The plots are representative of the average value obtained with different assays (n=6). The test conditions are described in Materials and Methods. FNB = phenobarbital unchanged

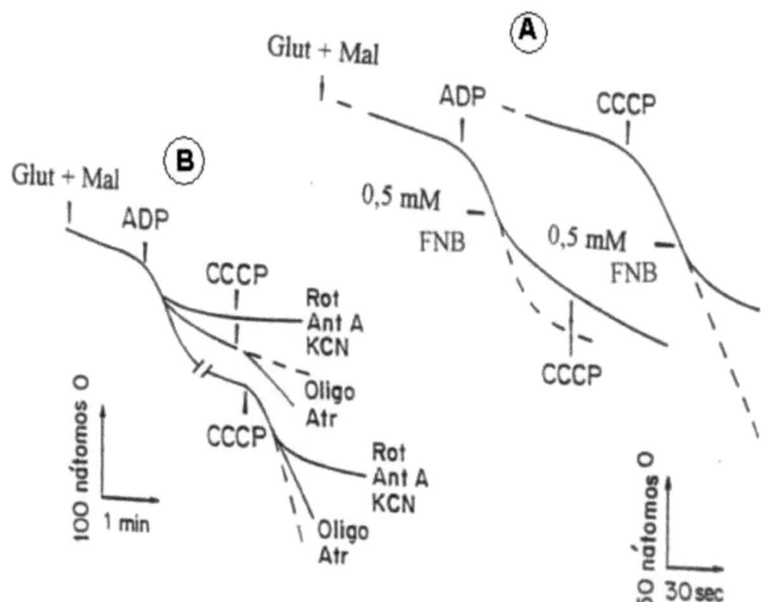

FIGURA 5 - (A): Effect of unchanged phenobarbital (FNB) on the respiration of rat liver mitochondria energized with 5 mM malate+ 5 mM glutamate, stimulated with ADP (0.4 μmol) or with the uncoupler CCCP (1 μg⁄ml). (B): Effect of rotenone (1μg⁄ml), antimycin A (1 μgZml), KCN (0.33 mM), oligomycin (1 μgZml), atractyloside (50 μm) and CCCP (0.1 μg⁄ml) (n=6). The test conditions are described in Materials and Methods. FNB = unchanged phenobarbital; CCCP= Carbonyl Cyanide P-Trichloromethoxyphenylhydrazone (uncoupler); Rot = rotenone; Ant A = antimycin A; Oligo = oligomycin; Atr = atractyloside.

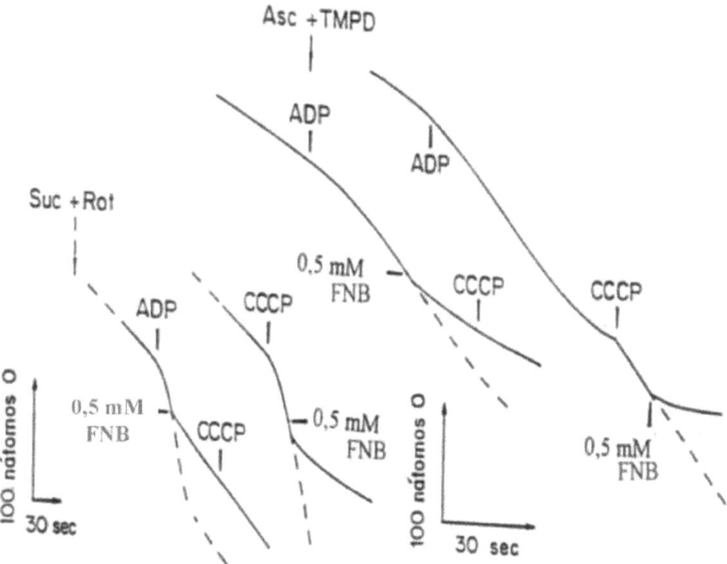

FIGURA 6 - Effect of unchanged phenobarbital (FNB) on the respiration of rat liver mitochondria energized with 10 mM succinate+ rotenone 1 μgZml or 4 mM ascorbate + 0.1 mM TMPD. Oxygen consumption in state 3 of respiration supported by succinate+ rotenone and ascorbate + TMPD are 142 and 184 n atoms of O/mg protein/min, respectively (n=6). The test conditions are described in Materials and Methods. FNB = unchanged phenobarbital; CCCP = chlorophenylhydrazone carbonyl cyanide (uncoupler).

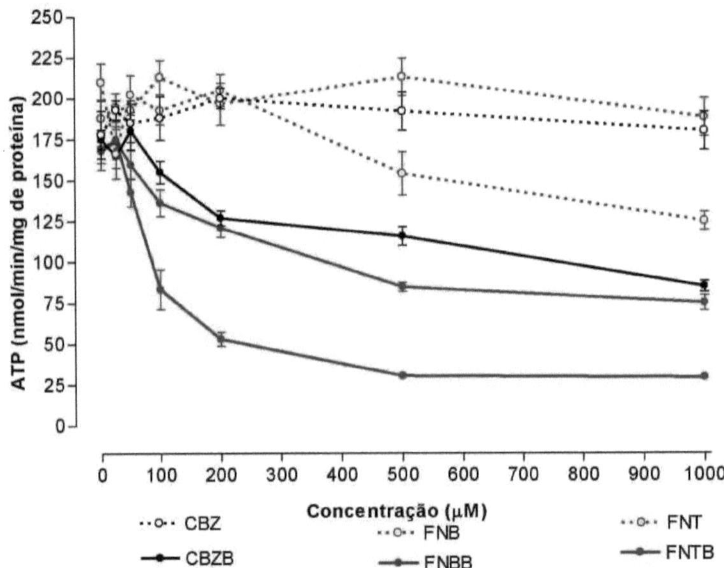

FIGURE 7 - Effects of unchanged and bioactivated drugs (carbamazepine, phenobarbital and phenytoin) on ATP synthesis (n=6). The test conditions are described in Materials and Methods. CBZ = unchanged carbamazepine; CBZB = bioactivated carbamazepine; FNB = unchanged phenobarbital; FNBB = bioactivated phenobarbital; FNT = phenytoin; FNTB = bioactivated phenytoin.

TABLE 2: Effects of carbamazepine, phenytoin and phenobarbital unchanged on MDA formation, GSH, GSSG, carbonyl protein (CP) and sulfhydryl protein (P-SH) levels in rat liver mitochondria.

	CBZ	**FNT**	**FNB**	**CONTROL POSITIVE (t-BOH)**	**CONTROL NEGATIVE**
MDA	5.0± 0.8	4.53± 0.57	4.2± 0.47	2.15± 0.63	4.50± 0.26
GSSG	0.046± 0.03	0,044±0,04	0.042± 0.01	0.059± 0.006	0.044± 0.03
GSH	0.70± 0.1	0.75± 0.37	0.74± 0.25	0.68± 0.43	0.73± 0.13
PC	98.0± 6.3	90± 5.4	95.0± 1.4	53.0± 3.5	95.0± 12.2
PSH	1.78± 0.3	1.81± 0.10	1.82± 0.07	4.75± 0.65	1.84± 0.09

t-BOH = t-butyl hydroperoxide; CBZ = carbamazepine unchanged; FNB = phenobarbital unchanged; FNT = phenytoin unchanged

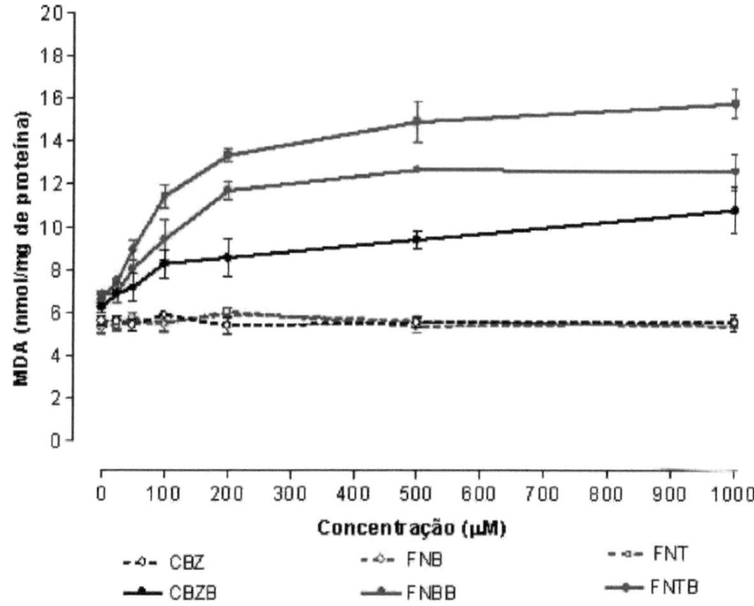

FIGURA 8. Effects of unchanged and bioactivated drugs (carbamazepine, phenobarbital and phenytoin) on mitochondrial malondialdehyde (MDA) levels (n=6). The assay conditions are described in Materials and Methods. CBZ = carbamazepine unchanged; CBZB = carbamazepine bioactivated; FNB = phenobarbital unchanged; FNBB = phenobarbital bioactivated; FNT = phenytoin; FNTB= phenytoin bioactivated

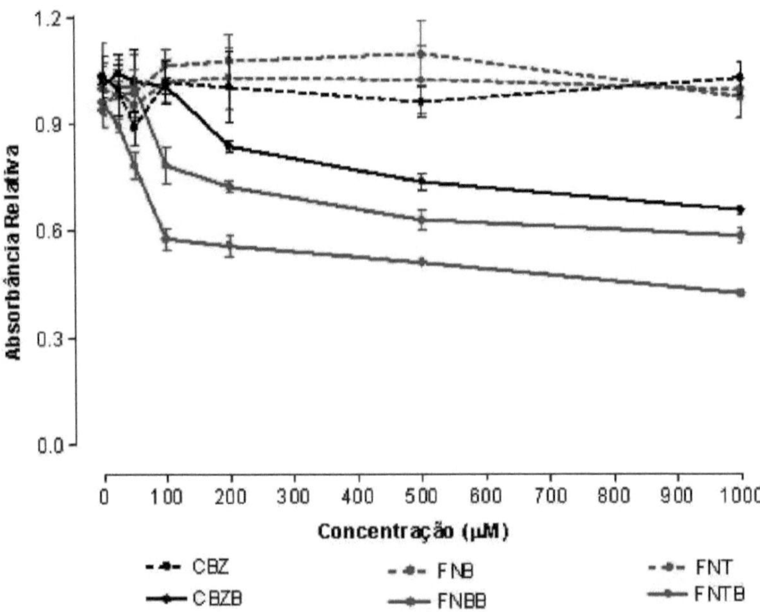

FIGURA 9. Effects of unchanged and bioactivated drugs (carbamazepine, phenobarbital and phenytoin) on mitochondrial cardiolipin levels (n=6). The assay conditions are described in Materials and Methods. CBZ = unchanged carbamazepine; CBZB = bioactivated carbamazepine; FNB = unchanged phenobarbital; FNBB = bioactivated phenobarbital; FNT = phenytoin; FNTB = bioactivated phenytoin.

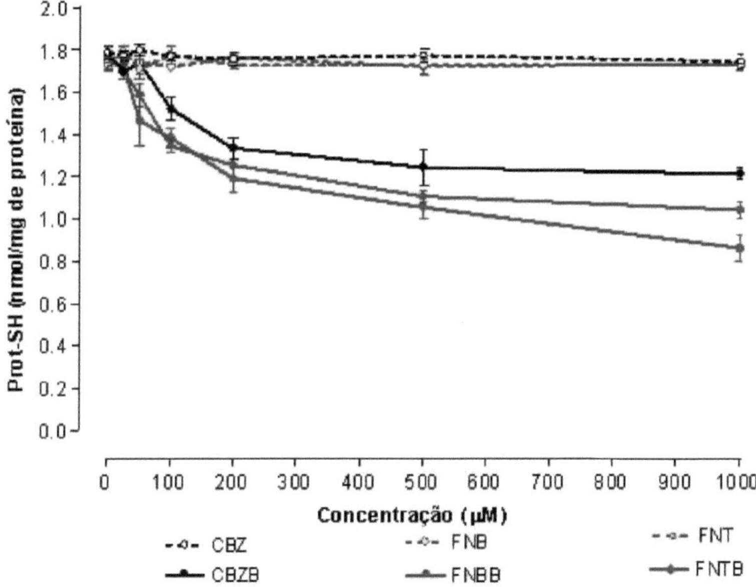

FIGURA 10. Effects of unchanged and bioactivated drugs (carbamazepine, phenobarbital and phenytoin) on mitochondrial sulfhydryl protein (Prot-SH) levels (n=6). The test conditions are described in Materials and Methods. CBZ = carbamazepine unchanged; CBZB = carbamazepine bioactivated; FNB = phenobarbital unchanged; FNBB = phenobarbital bioactivated; FNT = phenytoin; FNTB = phenytoin bioactivated.

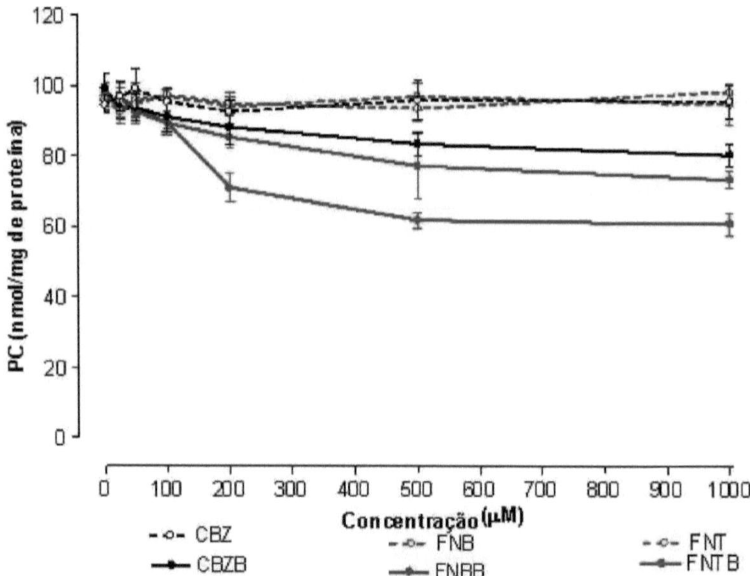

FIGURA 11. Effects of unchanged and bioactivated drugs (carbamazepine, phenobarbital and phenytoin) on mitochondrial protein carbonyl (PC) levels (n=6). The test conditions are described in Materials and Methods. CBZ = unchanged carbamazepine; CBZB = bioactivated carbamazepine; FNB = unchanged phenobarbital; FNBB = bioactivated phenobarbital; FNT = phenytoin; FNTB = bioactivated phenytoin.

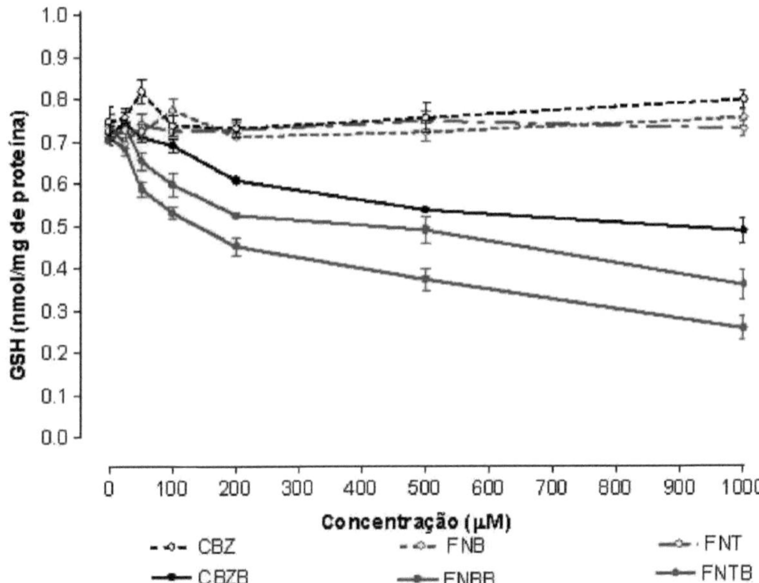

FIGURA 12. Effects of unchanged and bioactivated drugs (carbamazepine, phenobarbital and phenytoin) on mitochondrial reduced glutathione (GSH) levels (n=6). The test conditions are described in Materials and Methods. CBZ = carbamazepine unchanged; CBZB = carbamazepine bioactivated; FNB = phenobarbital unchanged; FNBB = phenobarbital bioactivated; FNT = phenytoin; FNTB = phenytoin bioactivated.

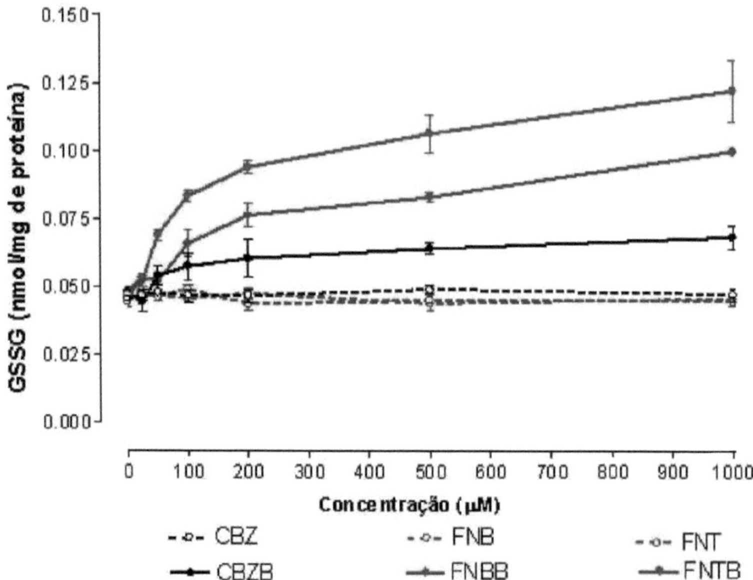

FIGURA 13. Effects of unchanged and bioactivated drugs (carbamazepine, phenobarbital and phenytoin) on mitochondrial oxidized glutathione (GSSG) levels (n=6). The test conditions are described in Materials and Methods. CBZ = carbamazepine unchanged; CBZB = carbamazepine bioactivated; FNB = phenobarbital unchanged; FNBB = phenobarbital bioactivated; FNT = phenytoin; FNTB = phenytoin bioactivated.

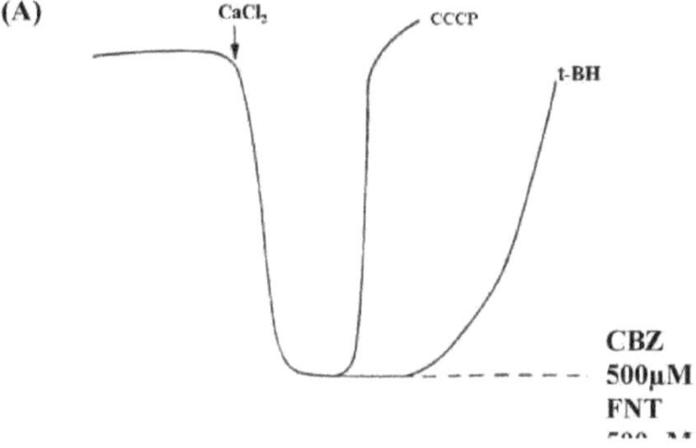

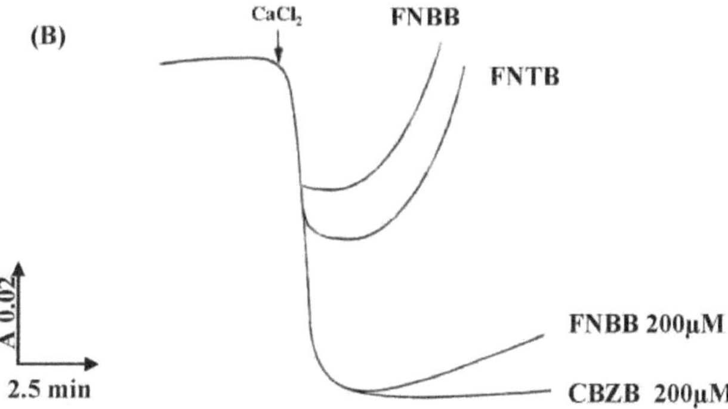

FIGURA 14. Effects of unchanged (A) and bioactivated (B) drugs (carbamazepine, phenobarbital and phenytoin) on calcium uptake and release (n=6). The test conditions are described in Materials and Methods. CBZ = unchanged carbamazepine; CBZB = bioactivated carbamazepine; FNB = unchanged phenobarbital; FNBB = bioactivated phenobarbital; FNT = phenytoin; FNTB = bioactivated phenytoin; t-BOOH= t-butyl hydroperoxide; CCCP = chlorophenylhydrazone carbonyl cyanide (uncoupler).

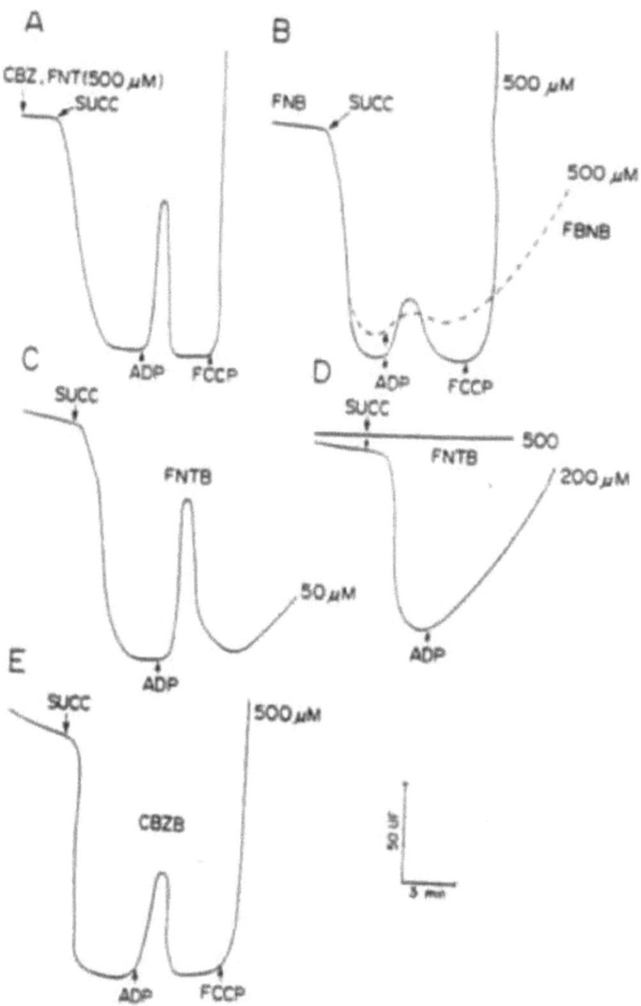

FIGURA 15. Effects of unchanged and bioactivated drugs (carbamazepine, phenobarbital and phenytoin) on mitochondrial membrane potential (n=6). The test conditions are described in Materials and Methods. CBZ = unchanged carbamazepine; CBZB = bioactivated carbamazepine; FNB = unchanged phenobarbital; FNBB = bioactivated phenobarbital; FNT = phenytoin; FNTB = bioactivated phenytoin.

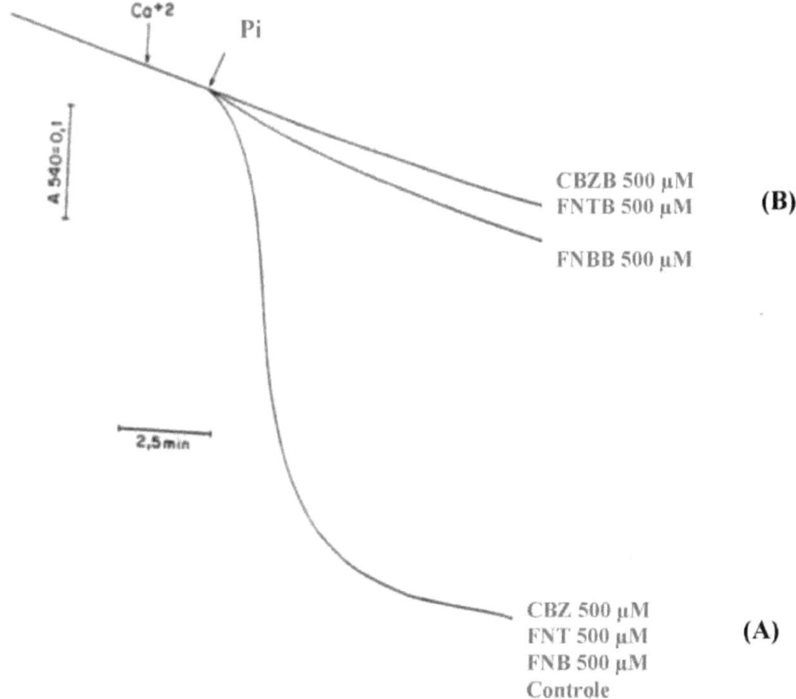

FIGURA 16. Effects of bioactivated drugs (carbamazepine, phenobarbital and phenytoin) on the swelling of rat liver mitochondria. The test conditions are described in Materials and Methods. CBZ = carbamazepine unchanged; CBZB = carbamazepine bioactivated; FNB = phenobarbital unchanged; FNBB = phenobarbital bioactivated; FNT = phenytoin; FNTB = phenytoin bioactivated.

DISCUSSION

The toxic effects of many drugs have been linked to their oxidation products, highly reactive electrophilic intermediate metabolites such as epoxides and areneoxides. The enzymes that catalyze this bioactivation vary according to the substrate and include the cytochrome P450 system, prostaglandin H synthase (PHS), and possibly lipooxygenases (LPOs). If these intermediates are not quickly neutralized by epoxide hydrolases and glutathione S-transferase (GST), their electrophilic centers (positively charged) can react with cellular constituents with electron-rich groups such as proteins, especially those containing thiol residues, forming a strong, irreversible covalent bond. If this covalent bond is not properly repaired, the adduct formed can initiate a process of cell damage, which can ultimately lead to cell death[130].

Another mechanism of toxic action of many drugs is the direct formation of a free radical and/or the subsequent indirect formation of reactive oxygen species (ROS) and the weakening of antioxidant defenses. The free radical derived directly from the drug can be centered on carbon, nitrogen or oxygen and has been associated with the toxic action (carcinogenicity, mutagenicity, cell necrosis and lipid peroxidation) of a wide variety of non-structurally related compounds. The free radical can be produced both enzymatically and non-enzymatically and, due to its high reactivity, can participate in a large number of reactions including: (1) electron transfer to molecular oxygen giving rise to superoxide anion and other reactive oxygen species; (2) hydrogen atom abstraction causing auto-oxidation of polyunsaturated fatty acids; and (3) covalent binding to macromolecules. ROS can oxidize diverse macromolecules such as proteins, lipids and DNA itself, a process known as oxidative stress [131].

There are two basic mechanisms by which drugs generate free radicals. The main one is the activation of drugs by the microsomal cytochrome P450 enzyme system. This system can metabolize molecules by making them free radicals through the addition of electrons (reduction), for example in the case of carbon tetrachloride and halothane; or by removing electrons (oxidation) 132. In the latter case, electron-deficient chemical species or electrophilic substances are formed. The products of these reactions may or may not be free radicals. Typical examples of drugs that are bioactivated by cytochrome P450 include acetaminophen and aromatic hydrocarbons, especially bromobenzene. The second mechanism of free radical formation occurs through the redox cycle, which does not necessarily involve the participation of cytochrome P-450[133,134].

Although they are relatively rare, idiosyncratic reactions are a major concern when starting therapy with AEs, and are the biggest cause of discontinuation of treatment with these drugs. Most AEA, including carbamazepine, phenytoin and phenobarbital, are predominantly metabolized in the liver, originating hydroxylated products formed through oxidations mediated by cytochrome P450. During this process, highly reactive intermediates known as areno-oxides are formed, which have a very short half-life and can cause damage to the sites of formation. The liver is therefore a particularly vulnerable organ to the toxicity of the highly reactive intermediate metabolites produced during biotransformation.

Areno-oxides are characterized by two double bonds in the aromatic ring which give them high reactivity, reacting rapidly with nucleophilic centers of cellular macromolecules such as DNA, RNA, proteins and lipids. The toxic, carcinogenic and mutagenic effects of aromatic compounds have often been correlated to the extent of their binding to biopolymers and there is strong evidence that arene oxides are the inducing agents of these effects. The extent to which arene oxides bind to cellular constituents depends on the speed with which they are formed as well as the speed with which they are converted into phenols, hydrated and conjugated with glutathione[26].

Antiepileptic-induced hepatotoxicity can occur as part of a generalized idiosyncratic reaction or as an isolated event, with a prevalence of around 9% among patients being treated with carbamazepine, phenytoin and phenobarbital [18,20].

The adverse reactions induced by AEA have been attributed to the accumulation of the arene oxides formed, which in turn can occur as a result of genetic or acquired metabolic deficiencies, such as deficiencies in the epoxide hydrolase enzyme, responsible for detoxifying these metabolites [84].

These idiosyncratic reactions have mainly been reported as immune-mediated; however, direct toxic effects can also occur. The cytotoxic effects of areno-oxides formed during the biotransformation of AEA have been previously evaluated by different authors through toxicity tests with human lymphocytes [26,83], but the role of mitochondria in the development of these effects has not yet been clarified.

In the present study, we evaluated the ability of AEA to alter mitochondrial function and promote oxidative stress, when subjected or not to the process of bioactivation with cytochrome P450 enzyme systems. Based on the method previously described by Spielberg et al. (1981)[27], the biotransformation of three classic AEA was carried out *in vitro* by the action of enzymes present *in* rat liver microsomes. This was the first study in the scientific literature to demonstrate the mitochondrial toxicity induced by these drugs and to outline the mechanisms involved. Until then, mitochondrial dysfunction had only been associated with hepatotoxicity induced by valproic acid, a non-aromatic antiepileptic drug[135].

The results found allow us to assume that mitochondrial dysfunction may be involved in both (1) idiosyncrasy associated with deficiencies of the epoxide hydrolase enzyme and (2) idiosyncrasy associated with genetic or acquired mitochondrial abnormalities. In the first case, there would be an accumulation of reactive metabolites which, in addition to acting as pro-hapten and initiating an immune response, as previously proposed[83], would also act by exerting a direct toxic effect on the liver mitochondria. In the second case, the accumulation of areno-oxides would not necessarily occur, but rather a greater mitochondrial susceptibility to the direct toxic effects of these metabolites, resulting in hepatocellular damage and death.

In fact, genetic or acquired mitochondrial abnormalities have been identified as the main factor determining susceptibility to a large number of drugs capable of affecting mitochondria and causing liver damage[136]. Our data strongly suggest that pre-existing mitochondrial abnormalities are factors that increase predisposition to idiosyncratic hepatotoxicity associated with the use of AEA.

In our study, mitochondrial energy metabolism was affected by the metabolites of the three AEA evaluated. As an unchanged drug (without bioactivation), only phenobarbital was able to affect mitochondrial function. Thus, with regard to mitochondrial dysfunction, the potency of the drugs studied was: activated phenytoin> activated phenobarbital> activated carbamazepine> unchanged phenobarbital. The other unchanged drugs had no effect on mitochondrial function.

The effect produced by phenobarbital only occurred at higher concentrations, but in the case of pre-existing liver disease this effect could become particularly important. Any impairment of liver function resulting in inhibition of biotransformation could cause accumulation of the unchanged drug and exacerbate its hepatotoxic effect.

At concentrations above 200 μM, phenobarbital caused a concentration-dependent and non-specific inhibition of electron transport. The pattern of inhibition of oxidative phosphorylation by phenobarbital showed the typical characteristics of site I (rotenone), site II (antimycin A) and site III (KCN) inhibitors of the respiratory chain. Phenobarbital inhibited respiration stimulated by both ADP and CCCP, indicating that both oxidative phosphorylation and electron transport were inhibited. In addition, state 3 inhibition occurred with different substrates, suggesting that complexes I, II and IV were probably affected, since malate/glutamate donate electrons to the respiratory chain via complex I, succinate via complex II and ascorbate/TMPD via complex IV. These data demonstrate a non-specific interaction of the unchanged drug with the components of the respiratory chain, with a consequent decrease in the flow of electrons at the three energy-conserving sites.

On the other hand, phenobarbital did not alter state 4 of respiration (respiration not activated by ADP), which suggests that the inner mitochondrial membrane remained intact. The effect of phenobarbital (unchanged) on mitochondrial function occurred only at high concentrations and, according to the indicators evaluated, was not mediated by oxidative stress, which explains the fact that the inner mitochondrial membrane was not damaged by the drug.

In contrast, all the bioactivated drugs inhibited respiration in state 3 and increased oxygen consumption in state 4, which suggests that as well as inhibiting electron transport, the metabolites of the three AEA also affected the inner mitochondrial membrane. In the specific case of phenobarbital, bioactivation intensified the effect on the respiratory chain, leading to inhibition at half the concentration (100 μM) when compared to the unchanged drug (200 μM). Such inhibition suggests that phenobarbital and particularly AEA metabolites can damage the respiratory chain and therefore interfere with energy metabolism. Confirming these findings, unchanged phenobarbital and all bioactivated drugs inhibited ATP synthesis.

Both unchanged phenobarbital and the bioactivated drugs affected the mitochondrial membrane potential, with bioactivation intensifying the effect of phenobarbital on this parameter. Bioactivated phenobarbital was ten times more effective (50 μM) in promoting this effect than the other bioactivated drugs (500 μM), which is in agreement with the findings regarding mitochondrial respiration and ATP synthesis. The mitochondrial membrane potential results from the efflux of protons from the matrix into the inter-membrane space and provides the energy required for ATP synthesis by complex V. Thus, based on its effect on electrochemical potential, it would be expected that bioactivated phenobarbital would be more effective in inhibiting ATP synthesis when compared to the unchanged drug.

In the case of calcium transport, only after bioactivation did the drugs show any effect. Consequently, inhibition of calcium-induced mitochondrial swelling also only occurred with bioactivated drugs. This is probably due to the mitochondria's inability to maintain the concentration of calcium necessary for the opening of the mitochondrial membrane permeability transition pore (MMPT) and the subsequent osmotic swelling of the organelle. In their unchanged form, the drugs were unable to induce/inhibit mitochondrial swelling or alter the uptake and release of calcium by the mitochondria.

Phenytoin, in particular, seems to have given rise to the metabolite with the greatest toxic potential, since lower concentrations of the bioactivated drug affected state 4 of respiration, RCR and ATP synthesis. In contrast, higher concentrations were required to inhibit state 3 of respiration, suggesting that the phenytoin metabolite acts primarily by causing structural damage to the inner mitochondrial membrane and not by directly inhibiting electron transfer.

The greater toxic effect of phenytoin can be attributed to extensive lipoperoxidation, as evidenced by indicators of oxidative stress and subsequent damage to the mitochondrial membrane. In fact, the initial increase observed in state 4 of respiration is consistent with this statement, since damage to the mitochondrial membrane normally leads to the uncoupling of mitochondrial respiration, given the mitochondria's difficulty in maintaining the electrochemical potential required to synthesize ATP. This greater effort is partially compensated for by increased oxygen consumption. Under normal conditions, around 2% of the oxygen used by the mitochondria does not undergo tetravalent reduction to H_2O and escapes from the electron transport chain in the form, mainly, of superoxide. The main point in the electron transport chain where this superoxide production occurs is the ubisemiquinone-cytochrome b region. The generation of ROS occurs mainly in state 4 of respiration, in the absence of ADP and in the presence of an excess of respiratory substrates. Under these conditions, the electron carriers are in a highly reduced state and it is possible that there is an increase in ubisemiquinone levels capable of reducing oxygen, causing an increase in ROS production. The generation of these ROS and their consequent interaction with free iron (Fenton reaction) results in the production of the hydroxyl radical ($OH^{\cdot}$). This chemical species is highly reactive and can attack biomolecular components and initiate lipoperoxidation of mitochondrial membranes, resulting in mitochondrial dysfunction[137,138].

The greater reactivity of the phenytoin metabolite could be explained by two factors: (1) the formation of a more reactive epoxide and/or (2) biotransformation on a larger scale. The first factor could be attributed to the more planar conformation of the molecule in which the epoxide group is more exposed and free to react. As for the second factor, it is known that, *in vivo,* phenytoin actually undergoes extensive biotransformation by the enzymes of the hepatic microsomal system, with over 95% of phenytoin being biotransformed in the liver and only 5% being eliminated unchanged in the urine[20]. It is known that an intermediate arene-oxide is formed during the conversion of phenytoin into the *para-hydroxyphenyl* phenytoin derivative (p-HPPH). This intermediate metabolite is thought to be involved in the idiosyncratic liver reactions associated with phenytoin, although this compound has never been isolated in plasma or urine, most likely due to its high instability [18].

Liver damage caused by phenytoin is rare, but fatal in 10 to 38% of cases [139]. The mechanism responsible for phenytoin hepatotoxicity has mainly been associated with hypersensitivity reactions involving the immune system [4,20,122]. Cytotoxicity has not yet been suggested as a mechanism for this event. Diwivedi et al. (2004) demonstrated a correlation between the toxicity of areno-oxides and phenytoin-induced skin rashes. Our data strongly suggest that cytotoxicity is also involved in phenytoin-induced hepatotoxicity and, furthermore, that mitochondrial dysfunction and oxidative stress are possible ways of mediating this toxic effect[140].

Among the bioactivated drugs, carbamazepine showed the least pronounced effects. A plausible explanation for this is the possibility that, compared to the other AEA studied, carbamazepine is biotransformed to a lesser extent by the hepatic microsomal system or that its biotransformation products are more rapidly metabolized to oxidized, more stable and less reactive products. The most important metabolite of carbamazepine, carbamazepine-10,11-epoxide, is pharmacologically active[20]. Its lower activity on mitochondria may be due to the fact that the epoxide group is protected by adjacent non-planar rings by a steric hindrance mechanism and is therefore less available to react compared to the planar phenytoin metabolite. Although stable, carbamazepine-10,11-epoxide can react covalently with macromolecules. In addition, carbamazepine hepatotoxicity has been correlated in some cases with another metabolite: carbamazepine-2,3-epoxide[18]. Two different types of carbamazepine-induced hepatotoxicity have been proposed: (1) hypersensitivity reaction and (2) toxin-induced reaction, both associated with the accumulation of areno-oxides and disturbances in glutathione metabolism [141]. The hypersensitivity reaction develops in the form of granulomatous hepatitis, with fever and abnormal liver function tests. The second type of liver damage results from direct drug toxicity and is characterized by acute hepatitis and hepatocellular necrosis, with fever, skin rashes and lymphadenopathy[20,13]9. The prognosis is usually favorable, and improvement is achieved with the cessation of treatment; however, fatal cases have been reported[142]. Our findings support the occurrence of liver damage caused by the direct toxic effect of metabolites from the biotransformation of carbamazepine and suggest that this toxic effect is on liver mitochondria. The profile of patients susceptible to carbamazepine-induced hepatotoxicity has not yet been established[20]. According to our findings, a possible susceptibility profile to carbamazepine and other AEA would be those individuals with mitochondrial abnormalities. Data from the scientific literature shows that the most frequent mitochondrial abnormalities in the general population are those related to alterations in complex I and complex IV of the respiratory chain[136,143]. Therefore, these individuals would be more predisposed to hepatotoxicity induced by drugs with mitochondrial toxicity, and according to our results, AEA is included in this group of drugs.

Cardiolipin is a phospholipid found mainly in the inner mitochondrial membrane and plays an important role in the structure and function of mitochondria[144]. Deficiency of this mitochondrial lipid has been associated with inhibition of state 3 of respiration and increased oxygen consumption in state 4, the latter of which seems to be associated with the production of ROS. Cardiolipin interacts with various proteins in the inner mitochondrial membrane and plays a central role in maintaining their activity. Among the proteins of the inner mitochondrial membrane are cytochrome oxidase, the ADP/ATP translocator, the phosphate translocator, substrate transporters, palmitoyl carnitine transferase/carnitine transferase systems and FoF1-ATPase. In addition, cardiolipin appears to play a central role in controlling the permeability of the inner mitochondrial membrane to small molecules, as well as in maintaining the mitochondrial proton gradient. Cardiolipin contains a high ratio of unsaturated to saturated fatty acids compared to other phospholipids in the inner mitochondrial membrane, a characteristic that makes it particularly sensitive to oxidative stress.[107,144] Our results show that cardiolipin was oxidized to a large extent by the bioactivated drugs, which may explain part of the effects observed.

One hypothesis that attempts to explain the mechanism involved in mitochondrial swelling proposes that this event depends on a decrease in mitochondrial membrane potential and is directly related to changes in sulfhydryl groups[14]5 . Another hypothesis proposes that the accumulation of ROS is due to the exhaustion of antioxidant defenses. ROS interact with sulfhydryl groups in mitochondrial membrane proteins, causing their oxidation and the opening of the permeability transition pore in the presence of calcium ion. Among the possible events that mediate the inhibition of pore opening are the direct interaction of the molecules with the pore, maintenance of the membrane potential, displacement of the calcium bond with cardiolipin and regeneration of the sulfhydryl groups[146]. As the oxidation of sulfhydryl groups is involved in mitochondrial swelling, we can speculate that the mitochondria were already swollen at the time of the test, hence the non-observance of the phenomenon. One piece of evidence for this claim is that during the mitochondrial swelling experiment, the absorbance observed was significantly lower in the bioactivation tests than in the controls carried out with the same protein concentration. This fact may also be related to the observation that mitochondria treated with bioactivated phenytoin and phenobarbital (200 µM) promoted calcium uptake, but were unable to retain the ion, releasing it afterwards. Richer et al. (1991) proposed that the combination of calcium and oxidative stress causes the activation of a specific mechanism for calcium efflux involving the hydrolysis of NADP to nicotinamide and ADP-ribose. Another possibility is that the release of calcium is the result of an increase in mitochondrial membrane permeability due to membrane damage caused by lipoperoxidation, particularly the oxidation of thiol groups in the inner mitochondrial membrane[147], which occurred to a great extent in our experimental model.

Based on the data obtained in this study, we could postulate two hypotheses for the mechanism of mitochondrial toxicity of the intermediate metabolites formed during the bioactivation of AEA:

(1) The metabolites would react covalently with the nucleophilic centers of the macromolecules critical for mitochondrial function and cause damage to the various mitochondrial membrane systems, resulting in the uncoupling of mitochondrial respiration (direct effect). This uncoupling would result in increased oxygen consumption and consequently greater generation of ROS, which would favor lipoperoxidation with additional damage to the mitochondrial membrane. In this context, lipoperoxidation would be the consequence of previous damage caused by the binding of arene oxides to mitochondrial macromolecules. The sum of these factors would lead the mitochondria to a total loss of its functional parameters, as was evident from the results presented;

(2) The metabolites react with the cisternae residues of glutathione, groups with which they have a high affinity. In the absence of catalase, the glutathione/glutathione peroxidase system is the mitochondria's main defense system against the ROS normally produced by the mitochondria. The

depletion of mitochondrial glutathione induced by bioactivated AEA and evidenced in our studies, could make mitochondria susceptible to lipoperoxidation with consequent oxidation of mitochondrial membrane constituents (indirect effect). The mitochondrion is an organelle whose function is entirely dependent on the integrity of the membrane systems and any alteration of a constituent of this system can have damaging consequences for its functioning. In this case, lipoperoxidation would act as a primary factor in the occurrence of the effects observed in mitochondrial function. Lipoperoxidation would compromise the various mitochondrial membrane systems, which would progressively, and depending on the concentration of the drugs and their respective biotransformation products, compromise mitochondrial function to such an extent that the mitochondria would become non-functional. This event was evidenced by the mitochondria's inability to respond to ADP, to form a membrane potential and consequently to undergo osmotic swelling. Furthermore, after the initial activation of state 4 (uncoupling), there was even inhibition of electron flow, particularly in the case of phenytoin, revealing a dysfunction in the electron carriers of the respiratory chain.

In short, our results strongly suggest that mitochondrial toxicity is one of the mechanisms involved in the idiosyncratic liver damage associated with treatment with AEA and occurs mainly due to the toxic effect of the metabolites produced by the action of liver enzymes during the biotransformation of these drugs. Thus, in addition to deficiencies in epoxide hydrolase, which have already been pointed out by other authors, mitochondrial abnormalities are also potential individual predisposing factors to the development of hepatotoxicity induced by AEA. Mitochondrial toxicity induced by these drugs has not previously been demonstrated in the scientific literature.

Given the widespread use of these drugs in the treatment of epilepsy, their recent and growing indication for the treatment of psychiatric and neurological disorders and the severity of their adverse effects, new strategies to protect against idiosyncratic reactions become necessary. In this context, the delineation of the possible mechanisms involved in AEA-induced hepatotoxicity could provide useful tools for the diagnosis, treatment and prevention of liver damage, which would contribute to the optimization of therapy with these drugs.

CONCLUSIONS

1. In the unchanged form, only phenobarbital affected mitochondrial function, without this effect being related to oxidative stress. State 3 of respiration induced by (a) pyruvate/malate, (b) succinate, or (c) ascorbate/TMPD was significantly inhibited, but there was no change in state 4. With regard to pyruvate/malate, the CI_{50} was 0.15 mM. The pattern of inhibition was similar to that exhibited by the respiratory chain inhibitors: rotenone, antimycin A and KCN. As a result, the membrane potential was also affected. Phenobarbital inhibited the rate of ATP synthesis in mitochondria energized with pyruvate/malate and depressed the phosphorylation potential.

(CI_{50} 0.2 mM). It was proposed that the inhibition of oxidative phosphorylation in rat mitochondria promoted by phenobarbital in its non-bioactivated form was due to the interaction of the drug with the mitochondrial membrane, more specifically on the components of the respiratory chain. These changes in the electron transport chain and oxidative phosphorylation were not able to induce significant changes in mitochondrial swelling or in the kinetics of calcium uptake and release.

2. When bioactivated, all the drugs had a marked effect on mitochondrial function and induced oxidative stress. The effects occurred at concentrations much lower than those observed for phenobarbital (around 50 μM). The order of potency of the bioactivated drugs was: phenytoin> phenobarbital> carbamazepine. Unlike phenobarbital, the bioactivation products of anticonvulsants had an uncoupling effect represented by an increase in baseline oxygen consumption (state 4 of respiration) with consequent repercussions on state 3 and RCR. Uncoupling is a clear sign of damage to the inner mitochondrial membrane. These effects are due to the intense oxidative stress observed, and the consequent oxidation of macromolecules (proteins and lipids, including cardiolipin), which are essential for maintaining the mitochondrial membrane systems. Particularly sensitive are proteins containing sulfhydryl groups, which are part of the catalytic site of many mitochondrial enzymes.

3. The mitochondrial toxicity exerted by metabolites from the hepatic biotransformation of AEA is probably one of the mechanisms involved in the idiosyncratic hepatotoxicity associated with the use of these drugs.

4. Pre-existing mitochondrial abnormalities, of genetic or acquired origin, are factors that possibly contribute to individual predisposition to AEA-induced hepatotoxicity.

REFERENCES

1 GODA K, KOBAYASHI A, TAKAHASHI A, TAKAHASHI T, SAITO K, MAEKAWA K, SAITO Y, SUGAI S.Evaluation of the Potential Risk of Drugs to Induce Hepatotoxicity in Human-Relationships between Hepatic Steatosis Observed in Non-Clinical Toxicity Study and Hepatotoxicity in Humans. Int J Mol Sci. 2017 Apr 12;18(4). pii: E810.

2 ALEMPIJEVIC T, ZEC S, MILOSAVLJEVIC T Drug-induced liver injury: Do we know everything?.World J Hepatol. 2017 Apr 8;9(10):491-502.

3 .LINDNER, A., et al. "Postinterventional pain and complications of sonographically guided interventions in the liver and pancreas." Ultraschall in der Medizin (Stuttgart, Germany: 1980) 35.2 (2014): 159.

4 KAPLOWITZ, N. Idiosyncratic drug hepatotoxicity. Nature Reviews. Drug Discovery, London, v. 4, p. 489-99, 2005.

5 .NAVARRO, V. J. and SENIOR, J. R. Drug-Related Hepatotoxicity, N Engl J Med; Boston, v. 354, p. 731-9, 2006

6 .JAMES, ROBERT C., and STEPHEN M. Roberts. "Hepatotoxicity: toxic effects on tHe Liver." Principles of Toxicology: Environmental and Industrial Applications (2014): 125.

7 PARK, B.K.; KITTERINGHAM, N.R.; MAGGS, J.L.; PIRMOHAMED, M.; WILLIAMS, D.P. The role of metabolic activation in drug-induced hepatotoxicity. Annual Review of Pharmacology and Toxicology Palo Alto, Calif.; v. 45, p. 177-202, 2005.

8 .WALGREN, J. L.; MITCHELL, M. D. and THOMPSON, D. C. " Role of Metabolism in Drug-Induced Idiosyncratic Hepatotoxicity", Critical Reviews in Toxicology, Boca Raton, v. 35, p. 325-361, 2005.

9 .UETRECHT, J., Idiosyncratic Drug Reactions: Current Understanding Annu Rev Pharmacol Toxicol. Palo Alto, Calif.; v. 47, p. 513-539, 2007.

10 .KENNA, J. GERRY. "Human biology-based drug safety evaluation: scientific rationale, current status and future challenges." Expert Opinion on Drug Metabolism & Toxicology 13.5 (2017): 567-574

11 .HOLT MP, JU C. Mechanisms of drug-induced liver injury. AAPS J 2006; 8: E48-E54

12 .SHEHU, AMINA IBRAHIM, XIAOCHAO MA, AND RAMAN VENKATARAMANAN. "Mechanisms of Drug-Induced Hepatotoxicity." Clinics in Liver Disease 21.1 (2017): 35-54. ;

13 KAPLOWITZ, N. Drug-Induced Liver Injury. Clinical Infectious Diseases, Los Angeles, v. 38,

Suppl 2, p. 44-48, 2004.

14 .SIES, HELMUT, CARSTEN BERNDT, and DEAN P. JONES. "Oxidative stress." Annual Review of Biochemistry 86.1 (2017). ;

15 .RECKNAGEL, R.O.; GLENDE, E.A.; BRITTON, R.S. Free Radical Damage and Lipid Peroxidation; in: MEEKS, R. G.; HARRISON, S.D.; BULL, R.J. Hepatology, Baltimore, p. 401-436, 1991.

16 .WELLS, P.G.; WINN, L.M. Biochemical toxicology of chemical teratogenesis. Critical Reviews in Biochemistry and Molecular Biology, Philadelphia, PA, v. 31, p. 1-40, 1996.Wells, P.G.; Winn, L.M.

17 .GOODMAN, ZACHARY D. "Phenotypes and Pathology of Drug-Induced Liver Disease." Clinics in Liver Disease 21.1 (2017): 89-101

18 ZACCARA, G.; FRANCIOTTA, D.; PERUCCA, E. Idiosyncratic adverse reactions to antiepileptic drugs. Epilepsia, New York, v. 48, p. 1223-1244, 2007.

19 COGNATO, G.D., BRUNO, A.N; DA SILVA, R.S.; BOGO, M.R.; SARKIS, J.J.; BONAN, C.D. Antiepileptic Drugs Prevent Changes Induced by Pilocarpine Model of Epilepsy in Brain Ecto-Nucleotidases. Neurochemical Research, New York, Plenum Press,

20 AHMED, S.N.; SIDDIQI, Z.A. Antiepileptic drugs and liver disease. Seizure, London v. 15, p. 156-164, 2006.

21 .ZWANZGER, P.; ESER, D.; RUPPRECHT, R. Anticonvulsants in the treatment of anxiety - an alternative treatment option? Nervenarzt, Berlin, v. 78, p. 1274-82, 2007.

22 NASREDDINE, W.; BEYDOUN, A. Oxcarbazepine in neuropathic pain. Expert Opinion on Investigational Drugs, London, v. 16, p. 1615-1625, 2007.

23 EISENBERG, E.; RIVER, Y.; SHIFRIN, A.; KRIVOY, N. Antiepileptic drugs in the treatment of neuropathic pain. Drugs, New York, v. 67, p. 1265-1289, 2007.

24 KAUFMAN, K.R.Comparative bioethics in bipolar and epilepsy research. Seizure. London : Baillière Tindall, v. 11, n. 1, p. 51-56, 2002.

25 PEYRIÈRE, H.; DEREURE, O.; BRETON, H.; DEMOLY, P.; COCIGLIO, M.; BLAYAC, J-P.; BUYS, D.H. Variability in the clinical pattern of cutaneous sideeffects of drugs with systemic symptoms: does a DRESS syndrome really exist? Therapeutiques, Paris, v. 155, p. 422-428, 2006.

26 BAVDEKAR, S.B.; MURANJAN, M.N.; GOGTAY, N.J.; KANTHARIA, V.; KSHIRSAGAR, N.A. Anticonvulsant hypersensitivity syndrome: lymphocyte toxicity assay for the confirmation of

diagnosis and risk assessment. The Annals of Pharmacotherapy, Cincinnati, OH, v. 38, p. 1648-1650, 2004.

27 SHEAR, N.H.; SPIELBERG, S.P. Anticonvulsant hypersensitivity syndrome. In vitro assessment of risk. The Journal of Clinical Investigation, New Haven, v. 82, p. 1826-1832, 1988.

28 FARRELL, G.C. Liver Disease Caused by Drugs, Anesthetics, and Toxins. In: Feldman M., Friedman L.S., Sleisenger M.H. (Eds.), Sleisenger & Fordtran's gastrointestinal and liver disease: pathophysiology, diagnosis, management. Elsevier, Philadelphia, p. 1411-1415, 2002.

29 .CHEN M, SUZUKI A, BORLAK J, ANDRADE RJ, LUCENA MI. Druginduced liver injury: Interactions between drug properties and host factors. J Hepatol 2015; 63: 503-514

30 FISHER K, VUPPALANCHI R, SAXENA R. Drug-Induced Liver Injury. Arch Pathol Lab Med 2015; 139: 876-887

31 CHEN M, BORLAK J, TONG W. High lipophilicity and high daily dose of oral medications are associated with significant risk for drug-induced liver injury. Hepatology 2013; 58: 388-396

32 CHEN M, TUNG CW, SHI Q, GUO L, SHI L, FANG H, BORLAK J, TONG W. A testing strategy to predict risk for drug-induced liver injury in humans using high-content screen assays and the 'rule-of-two' model. Arch Toxicol 2014; 88: 1439-1449

33 .BOELSTERLI UA, LEE PK. Mechanisms of isoniazid-induced idiosyncratic liver injury: emerging role of mitochondrial stress. J Gastroenterol Hepatol 2014; 29: 678-687

34 MAYORAL W, LEWIS JH, ZIMMERMAN H. Drug-induced liver disease. Curr Opin Gastroenterol 1999; 15: 208-216

35 LEWIS JH. The Art and Science of Diagnosing and Managing Drug-induced Liver Injury in 2015 and Beyond. Clin Gastroenterol Hepatol 2015; 13: 2173-2189.e8

36.OSTAPOWICZ G, FONTANA RJ, SCHI0DT FV, LARSON A, DAVERN TJ, HAN SH, MCCASHLAND TM, SHAKIL AO, HAY JE, HYNAN L, CRIPPIN JS, BLEI AT, SAMUEL G, REISCH J, LEE WM. Results of a prospective study of acute liver failure at 17 tertiary care centers in the United States. Ann Intern Med 2002; 137: 947-954

37 LEE WM. Drug-induced acute liver failure. Clin Liver Dis 2013; 17: 575-586, viii

38 .REUBEN A, KOCH DG, LEE WM. Drug-induced acute liver failure: results of a U.S. multicenter, prospective study. Hepatology 2010; 52: 2065-2076

39 LEWIS JH. Drug-induced liver injury throughout the drug development life cycle: where we have been, where we are now and where we are headed - perspectives of a clinical hepatologist.

Pharm Med 2013; 27: 165-191

40 . AVIGAN MI. DILI and drug development: a regulatory perspective. Semin Liver Dis 2014; 34: 215-226

41 REGEV A. Drug-induced liver injury and drug development: industry perspective. Semin Liver Dis 2014; 34: 227-239

42 SENIOR JR. Evolution of the Food and Drug Administration approach to liver safety assessment for new drugs: current status and challenges. Drug Saf 2014; 37 Suppl 1: S9-17

43 .GUO T, GELPERIN K, SENIOR JR. A tool to help you decide (detect potentially serious liver injury). [accessed 2016 Aug 11]. Available from: URL: https://www.fda.gov/downloads/Drugs/Science

Research/ResearchAreas/ucm076777.pdf],

44 .BRINKER AD, LYNDLY J, TONNING J, MOENY D, LEVINE JG, AVIGAN MI. Profiling cumulative proportional reporting ratios of druginduced liver injury in the FDA Adverse Event Reporting System (FAERS) database. Drug Saf 2013; 36: 1169-1178

45 BEHRMAN RE, BENNER JS, BROWN JS, MCCLELLAN M, WOODCOCK J, PLATT R. Developing the Sentinel System--a national resource for evidence development. N Engl J Med 2011; 364: 498-499

46 .CHEN M, ZHANG J, WANG Y, LIU Z, KELLY R, ZHOU G, FANG H, BORLAK J, TONG W. The liver toxicity knowledge base: a systems approach to a complex end point. Clin Pharmacol Ther 2013; 93: 409-412

47 .FELSER A, BLUM K, LINDINGER PW, BOUITBIR J, KRÀHENBÜHL S. Mechanisms of hepatocellular toxicity associated with dronedarone- -a comparison to amiodarone. Toxicol Sci 2013; 131: 480-490

48 ANDREWS S, HOLDEN R. Characteristics and management of immunerelated adverse effects associated with ipilimumab, a new immunotherapy for metastatic melanoma. Cancer Manag Res 2012; 4: 299-307

49 KLEINER DE, BERMAN D. Pathologic changes in ipilimumabrelated hepatitis in patients with metastatic melanoma. Dig Dis Sci 2012; 57: 2233-2240

50 .STINE JG, LEWIS JH. Drug-induced liver injury: a summary of recent advances. Expert Opin Drug Metab Toxicol 2011; 7: 875-890

51 .WATKINS PB, LEWIS JH, KAPLOWITZ N, ALPERS DH, BLAIS JD, SMOTZER DM,

KRASA H, OUYANG J, TORRES VE, CZERWIEC FS, ZIMMER CA. Clinical Pattern of Tolvaptan-Associated Liver Injury in Subjects with Autosomal Dominant Polycystic Kidney Disease: Analysis of Clinical Trials Database. Drug Saf 2015; 38: 1103-1113

52 MARTINEZ MA, VUPPALANCHI R, FONTANA RJ, STOLZ A, KLEINER DE, HAYASHI PH, GU J, HOOFNAGLE JH, CHALASANI N. Clinical and histologic features of azithromycin-induced liver injury. Clin Gastroenterol Hepatol 2015; 13: 369-376.e3

53 .VUPPALANCHI R, HAYASHI PH, CHALASANI N, FONTANA RJ, BONKOVSKY H, SAXENA R, KLEINER D, HOOFNAGLE JH. Duloxetine hepatotoxicity: a case-series from the drug-induced liver injury network. Aliment Pharmacol Ther 2010; 32: 1174-1183

54 .ORMAN ES, CONJEEVARAM HS, VUPPALANCHI R, FRESTON JW, ROCHON J, KLEINER DE, HAYASHI PH. Clinical and histopathologic features of fluoroquinolone- induced liver injury. Clin Gastroenterol Hepatol 2011; 9: 517-523.e3

55 .RUSSO MW, HOOFNAGLE JH, GU J, FONTANA RJ, BARNHART H, KLEINER DE, CHALASANI N, BONKOVSKY HL. Spectrum of statin hepatotoxicity: experience of the drug-induced liver injury network. Hepatology 2014; 60: 679-686

56 .BRINKER AD, WASSEL RT, LYNDLY J, SERRANO J, AVIGAN M, LEE WM, SEEFF LB. Telithromycin-associated hepatotoxicity: Clinical spectrum and causality assessment of 42 cases. Hepatology 2009; 49: 250-257

1. IACOVELLI R, PALAZZO A, PROCOPIO G, SANTONI M, TRENTA P, DE BENEDETTO A, MEZI S, CORTESI E. Incidence and relative risk of hepatic toxicity in patients treated with anti-angiogenic tyrosine kinase inhibitors for malignancy. Br J Clin Pharmacol 2014; 77: 929-938

58. CHALHOUB WM, SLIMAN KD, ARUMUGANATHAN M, LEWIS JH. Druginduced liver injury: what was new in 2013? Expert Opin Drug Metab Toxicol 2014; 10: 959-980

59. DALY AK, DAY CP. Genetic association studies in drug-induced liver injury. Drug Metab Rev 2012; 44: 116-126

60. URBAN TJ, DALY AK, AITHAL GP. Genetic basis of drug-induced liver injury: present and future. Semin Liver Dis 2014; 34: 123-133

61. CHEN R, ZHANG Y, TANG S, LV X, WU S, SUN F, XIA Y, ZHAN SY. The association between HLA-DQB1 polymorphism and antituberculosis drug-induced liver injury: a Case-Control Study. J Clin Pharm Ther 2015; 40: 110-115

62. VISSCHERS RG, LUYER MD, SCHAAP FG, OLDE DAMINK SW, SOETERS PB. The gut-liver axis. Curr Opin Clin Nutr Metab Care 2013; 16: 576-581

63. POSSAMAI LA, MCPHAIL MJ, KHAMRI W, WU B, CONCAS D, HARRISON M, WILLIAMS R, COX RD, COX IJ, ANSTEE QM, THURSZ MR. The role of intestinal microbiota in murine models of acetaminophen-induced hepatotoxicity. Liver Int 2015; 35: 764-773

64. HAWKINS MT, LEWIS JH. Latest advances in predicting DILI in human subjects: focus on biomarkers. Expert Opin Drug Metab Toxicol 2012; 8: 1521-1530

65. BELL LN, VUPPALANCHI R, WATKINS PB, BONKOVSKY HL, SERRANO J, FONTANA RJ, WANG M, ROCHON J, CHALASANI N. Serum proteomic profiling in patients with drug-induced liver injury. Aliment Pharmacol Ther 2012; 35: 600-612

66. STEUERWALD NM, FOUREAU DM, NORTON HJ, ZHOU J, PARSONS JC, CHALASANI N, FONTANA RJ, WATKINS PB, LEE WM, REDDY KR, STOLZ A, TALWALKAR J, DAVERN T, SAHA D, BELL LN, BARNHART H, GU J, SERRANO J, BONKOVSKY HL. Profiles of serum cytokines in acute drug-induced liver injury and their prognostic significance. PLoS One 2013; 8: e81974 [DOI: 10.1371/journal.pone.0081974];

67. WELCH MA, KOCK K, URBAN TJ, BROUWER KL, Swaan PW. Toward predicting drug-induced liver injury: parallel computational approaches to identify multidrug resistance protein 4 and bile salt export pump inhibitors. Drug Metab Dispos 2015; 43: 725-734

68. ALEO MD, LUO Y, SWISS R, BONIN PD, POTTER DM, WILL Y. Human drug- induced liver injury severity is highly associated with dual inhibition of liver mitochondrial function and bile salt export pump. Hepatology 2014; 60: 1015-1022

69. RIBEIRO MP, SANTOS AE, CUSTÓDIO JB. Mitochondria: the gateway for tamoxifen-induced liver injury. Toxicology 2014; 323: 10-18

70. WEBB GJ, ADAMS DH. Modeling idiosyncrasy: a novel animal model of drug-induced liver injury. Hepatology 2015; 61: 1124-1126

71. METUSHI IG, CAI P, ZHU X, NAKAGAWA T, UETRECHT JP. A fresh look at the mechanism of isoniazid-induced hepatotoxicity. Clin Pharmacol Ther 2011; 89: 911-914

72. FONTANA RJ. Pathogenesis of idiosyncratic drug-induced liver injury and clinical perspectives. Gastroenterology 2014; 146: 914-928

73. ROCKEY DC, SEEFF LB, ROCHON J, FRESTON J, CHALASANI N, BONACINI M, FONTANA RJ, HAYASHI PH. Causality assessment in drug-induced liver injury using a structured expert opinion process: comparison to the Roussel-Uclaf causality assessment method. Hepatology 2010; 51: 2117-2126

74. LEWIS JH. Causality assessment: which is best-expert opinion or RUCAM? Clinical Liver Dis

2014; 4: 4-8

75. REGEV A, SEEFF LB, MERZ M, ORMARSDOTTIR S, AITHAL GP, GALLIVAN J, WATKINS PB. Causality assessment for suspected DILI during clinical phases of drug development. Drug Saf 2014; 37 Suppl 1: S47-S56

76. TEO YL, HO HK, CHAN A. Formation of reactive metabolites and management of tyrosine kinase inhibitor-induced hepatotoxicity: a literature review. Expert Opin Drug Metab Toxicol 2015; 11: 231-242

77. MOMEN-HERAVI F, BALA S, BUKONG T, SZABO G. Exosomemediated delivery of functionally active miRNA-155 inhibitor to macrophages. Nanomedicine 2014; 10: 15171527

78. LEXMOND WS, VAN DAEL CM, SCHEENSTRA R, GOORHUIS JF, SIEDERS E, VERKADE HJ, VAN RHEENEN PF, KOMHOFF M. Experience with molecular adsorbent recirculating system treatment in 20 children listed for high-urgency liver transplantation. Liver Transpl 2015; 21: 369-380

79. LIU CT, CHEN TH, CHENG CY. Successful treatment of druginduced acute liver failure with high-volume plasma exchange. J Clin Apher 2013; 28: 430-434

80. WREE A, DECHÊNE A, HERZER K, HILGARD P, SYN WK, GERKEN G, CANBAY A. Steroid and ursodeoxycholic acid combination therapy in severe drug-induced liver injury. Digestion 2011; 84: 54-59

81. SINGH S, HYNAN LS, LEE WM. Improvements in hepatic serological biomarkers are associated with clinical benefit of intravenous N-acetylcysteine in early stage nonacetaminophen acute liver failure. Dig Dis Sci 2013; 58: 1397-1402

82. SQUIRES RH, DHAWAN A, ALONSO E, NARKEWICZ MR, SHNEIDER BL, RODRIGUEZ-BAEZ N, OLIO DD, KARPEN S, BUCUVALAS J, LOBRITTO S, RAND E, ROSENTHAL P, HORSLEN S, NG V, SUBBARAO G, KERKAR N, RUDNICK D, LOPEZ MJ, SCHWARZ K, ROMERO R, ELISOFON S, DOO E, ROBUCK PR, LAWLOR S, BELLE SH. Intravenous N-acetylcysteine in pediatric patients with nonacetaminophen acute liver failure: a placebo-controlled clinical trial. Hepatology 2013; 57: 1542-1549

83. BOHAN, K.H.; MANSURI, T.F.; WILSON, N.M. Anticonvulsant hypersensitivity syndrome: implications for pharmaceutical care. Pharmacotherapy, Boston, MA., v. 27, p. 1425-1439, 2007.

84. SIERRA, N.M.; GARCIA, B.; MARCO, J.; PLAZA, S.; HIDALGO, F.; BERMEJO, T. Cross hypersensitivity syndrome between phenytoin and carbamazepine. Pharmacy World & Science, The Hague, v. 27, p. 170-174, 2005.

85. WELLS, P. G.; BHULLERA, Y.; CHENA, C. S.; JENGA, W.; KASAPINOVICA, S.; K ENNEDYA, J. C.; KIMA, P. M.; LAPOSA, R. R.; MCCALLUMA, G. P.; NICOLB, C. J.; PARMANA, T.;MICHAEL, J.; WILEYC; WONGA, A. W. Molecular and biochemical mechanisms in teratogenesis involving reactive oxygen species. Toxicology and Applied Pharmacology, New York, v. 207, p. S354- S366, 2005.

86. DENNERY, P. A. Effects of Oxidative Stress on Embryonic Development, Birth Defects Research (Part C), Hoboken, NJ, v. 81, p. 155-162, 2007.

87. GOLDSTEIN, R.S.; SCHELLMANN. Toxic Response of the Kidney; In: KLAASSEN, C.D. CASARETT and DOULL'S. Toxicology. The Basis of Poisons. 5 ed., Mc Graw-Hill, Inc., New York, p. 417-443, 1994.

88. EKOUE DN, HE C, DIAMOND AM, BONINI MG. Manganese superoxide dismutase and glutathione peroxidase-1 contribute to the rise and fall of mitochondrial reactive oxygen species which drive oncogenesis. Biochim Biophys Acta. 2017 Jan 11. pii: S0005- 2728(17)30007-5.

89. CERVINKOVA, Z.; LOTKOVA, H.; KRIVAKOVA, P.; ROUSAR, T.; KUCERA, O.; TICHY, L.; CERVINKA, M.; DRAHOTA, Z., Evaluation of mitochondrial function in isolated rat hepatocytes and mitochondria during oxidative stress. Altern Lab Anim., London, v. 35, n. 3, p. 353-361, 2007.

90. XIONGA, J.; CAMELLO, P.J.; VERKHRATSKY, A.; TOESCU , E. C.Mitochondrial polarization status and [Ca2+]i signalling in rat cerebellar granule neurons aged in vitro, Neurobiol Aging, Fayetteville, N.Y., v. 25, n. 3, p. 349-359, 2004.

91. KARPLUS, M.; YI QIN GAO; JIANPENG, M.A.; ARJAN, V.D. V. AND W, Y., Protein structural transitions and their functional role, Phil. Trans. R. Soc. A, London, v. 363, p. 331356, 2005.

92. REINDERS, J.; WAGNER, K.; RENE, P.; ZAHEDI, D.; STOJANOVSKI, B. E.; VAN DER LAAN, M.;, REHLING, P.; SICKMANN, A.; PFANNER, N. AND MEISINGER, C. Profiling phosphoproteins of yeast mitochondria reveals a role of phosphorylation in assembly of the ATP synthase, Downloaded from ww.mcponline.org at CAPES Usage on October 11, 2007 www.mcponline.org Downloaded , MCP Papers in Press. Published on August 29, 2007 as Manuscript M700098-MCP200, 2007.

93. GÓMEZ-PUYOU, A.; SAAVEDRA-LIRA, E.; BECKER, I.; ZUBILLAGA, R.A.; ROJO-DOMiNGUEZ, A.; PÉREZ-MONTFORT, R. Using evolutionary changes to achieve speciesspecific inhibition of enzyme action--studies with triosephosphate isomerase. Chem Biol., London, v. 2, n. 12, p. 847-855,1995.

94. YAGUZHINSKY, L. S.; VLADIMIR, I.; YURKOV, I. P.; KRASINSKAYA On the localized coupling of respiration and phosphorylation in mitochondria. Biochimica et Biophysica Acta, Amsterdam, v. 1757, p. 408-414, 2006.

95. CAVANAGH, F.; INSERRA, M.; FERDER, L., From Mitochondria to Disease: Role of the Renin-Angiotensin System Am J Nephrol., Basel ; New York : Karger, v. 27, p. 545-553, 2007.

96. VERCESI, A.E.; Dissociation of NAD(P)+-stimulated mitochondrial Ca2+ efflux from swelling and membrane damage. Arch. of Biochem. Biophys., New York, NY, v. 232, p. 8691, 1984.

97. ROSCA, M. G.; MUSTATA, T.G.; KINTER, M. T.; OZDEMIR, A.M.; KERN, T. S.; SZWEDA, L. I.; BROWNLEE, M.; MONNIER, V. M. AND WEISS, M.F. Glycation of mitochondrial proteins from diabetic rat kidney is associated with excess superoxide formation . Am J Physiol Renal Physiol., Bethesda, v. 289, p. F420-F430, 2005.

98. GRIVENNIKOVA, V. G., ANDREI D. VINOGRADOV , Generation of superoxide by the mitochondrial Complex I., Biochimica et Biophysica Acta., Amsterdam, v. 1757, p. 553561, 2006.

99. CASADEMONT, J.; GARRABOU, G.; MIRO, O.; LOPEZ, S.; PONS, A.; BERNARDO, M.; CARDELLACH, F., Neuroleptic Treatment Effect on Mitochondrial Electron Transport Chain: Peripheral Blood Mononuclear Cells Analysis in Psychotic Patients. Journal of Clinical Psychopharmacology, Baltimore, Md, v. 27, n. 3, p. 284-288, 2007.

100. TALLMAN, J.F.; PAUL, S.M.; SKOLNICK, P.; GALLAGER, D.W. Receptors for the age of anxiety: pharmacology of the benzodiazepines. Science. New York; v. 207, n. 4428,p. 274-281, 1980.

101. VERMA, A.; SNYDER, S.H. Peripheral type benzodiazepine receptors. Annu Rev Pharmacol Toxicol. Palo Alto, Calif.; v. 29, p. 307-22, 1989.

102. CODE, W.D.; WHITE, H,S.; HERTZ, L. The effect of midazolam on calcium signaling in atrocytes. Ann. N. Y. Sci., New York, v. 625, p. 430-432, 1991.

103. YANAGIBASHI, K.; OHNO, Y.; NAKAMICHI, N.; MATSUI, T.; HAYASHIDA, K.; TAKAMURA, M.; YAMADA, K.; TOU, S.; KAWAMURA. M. Peripheral-type benzodiazepine receptors are involved in the regulation of cholesterol side chain cleavage in adrenocortical mitochondria. J Biochem, Tokyo, v. 106, n. 6, p. 1026-1029, 1989.

104. HIRSCH, J.D.; BEYER, F.; MALKOWITZ,L.; BEER, B.; BLUME, A.J. Mitochondrial benzodiazepine receptors mediate inhibition of mitochondrial respiratory control. Mol Pharmacol., New York, v. 34, p. 157-163, 1988.

105. VALKO, M.; RHODES, C.J.; MONCOL, J.; IZAKOVIC, M.; MAZUR, M. Free radicals, metals and antioxidants in oxidative stress-induced cancer. Chem Biol Interact, Elsevier, v. 160, n. 1,

p. 1-40, 2006.

106. OLIVER, C.N.; STARKE-REED, B.; STADMAN,E.R.; LIU, G.J.; CARNEY, J.M.; FLOYD, R.A. Oxidative damage on glutamine synthetase activity, and production of free radicals during eschemia reperfusion-induced injuries to gerbil brain. Proc. Natl. Acad. Sci., Washington, v. 87, p. 5144-47, 1990.

107. HAUFF, K. D.; HATCH, G. M. Cardiolipin metabolism and Barth Syndrome. Prog. Lipid Res., Elmsford, v. 45, n. 2, p. 91-101, 2006.

108. OLIVEIRA, M. R., MOREIRA, J. C. F., Acute and chronic vitamin A supplementation at therapeutic doses induces oxidative stress in submitochondrial particles isolated from cerebral cortex and cerebellum of adult rats. Toxicology Letters, Elsevier, v. 173, p. 145-150, 2007.

109. HALLIWELL, B.; GUTTERIDGE, J.M.C. Protection against oxidants in biological systems: The superoxide theory of oxygen toxicity. in: Halliwell, B.; Gutteridge, J.M.C. Free Radical in Biological and Medicine. Clarendon Press, p. 86, 1989.

110. MEHROTRA, S.; KAKKAR, P.; VISWANATHAN, P.N. Mitochondrial damage by active oxygen species in vitro. Free Radic Biol Med. New York : Pergamon v. 10, n. 5, p. 277-285,1991.

111. VERCESI, A.E.; HOFFMANN, M.E. Generation of reactive oxygen metabolites and oxidative damage in mitochondria: The role of calcium. In: JONES, D.P.; LASH, L.H. (eds.). Methods in toxicology, Academic Press, New York, p. 256-265, 1993.

112. BENZI, G.; MORETTI, A. Age-and peroxidative stress-related modifications of the cerebral enzymatic activities linked to mitochondria and the gluthathione system. Free Radic Biol Med. New York, v. 19, p. 77-101, 1995.

113. JENNER, P. Oxidative damage in neurodegenerative disease. Lancet, London, v. 344, p. 769-778, 1994.

114. CHOI, J.; HOWARD, D.; REES, S.T.; WEINTRAUB, A.I.; LEVEY; CHIN, L.-S. AND LI, L., Oxidative Modifications and Aggregation of Cu,Zn-Superoxide Dismutase Associated with Alzheimer and Parkinson Diseases The Journal Of Biological Chemistry, Baltimore, v. 280, n. 12, Issue of March 25, p. 11648-11655, 2005.

115. TRUMP, B.F.; BEREZESKY, I.K. Calcium-mediated cell injury and cell death. Faseb J., Bethesda, v. 9, p. 219-228, 1995.129.Zima, 2003).

116. LITSKY, M.L.; PFEIFFER, D.R. Regulation of the mitochondrial Ca2+ uniporter by external adenine nucleotides: The uniporter behaves like a gated channel that is regulated by nucleotides and divalent cations. Biochemistry, Washington, v. 36, p. 7071 - 7080, 1997

117. CASTILHO, R.F.; KOWALTOWSKI, A.J.; VERCESI, A.E. The irreversibility of inner mitochondrial membrane permeabilization by Ca2+ plus prooxidants is determined by the extent of membrane protein thiol cross-linking. J. Bioenerg. Biomembr., New York, v. 28, n. 6, p. 523-529, 1996.

118. BABCOCK, D.F.; HERRINGTON, J.; GOODWIN, P.C.; PARK, Y.B.; HILLE, B. Mitochondrial participation in the cellular Ca2+ network. J.Cell Biol, New York, v. 136, n. 4, p. 833 -844, 1997.

119. LEMASTERS, J.J.; NIEMINEN, A-L.; QIAN, T.; TROST, L.C.; HERMAN, B. The mitochondrial permeability transition toxic, hypoxic and reperfusion injury. Mol. and Cell. Biochem., Kluwer Academic, Netherlands, v. 174, p. 159-165, 1997.

120. PEREIRA, R.S.; BERTOCCHI, A.P.F.; VERCESI, A.E. Protective effect of trifluoperazine on the mitochondrial damage induced by Ca2+ plus prooxidants. Biochemical Pharmacology, Oxford, v. 24, p. 1795-1801, 1992.

121. LEHNINGER, A.L.; REYNAFARJE, B.; VERCESI, A.; TEW, W.P. Transport and accumulation of calcium in mitochondria. Ann N Y Acad Sci, New York, NY, v. 28, n. 307, p. 160-176, 1978.

122. KASS, G.E. Mitochondrial involvement in drug-induced hepatic injury. Chemical Biological Interactions, Elsevier, v. 163, p. 145-159, 2006.

123. MARTIN, C.N.; GARNER, R.C. The identification and assessment of covalent binding in vitro and in vivo. In: Snell K, Mullock B (Eds). Biochemical Toxicology: a practical approach. IRL Press, Oxford, p. 109-126, 1987.

124. ESTABROOK, R.W. Mitochondrial respiratory control and the polarographic measurement of ADP: O ratios. Methods Enzymol. New York v. 10, p. 41-47, 1967.

125. EMAUS, R. K.; GRUNWALD, R.; LEMASTERS, J. J. Rhodamine-123 as a probe of transmembrane potential in isolated rat-liver mitochondria - spectral and metabolic properties. Biochimica et Biophysica Acta, Amsterdam, v. 850,p. 436-48, 1986.

126. BUEGE, J.A.; AUST, S.D. Microsomal lipid peroxidation. Gleischer, S.; Packer, L. In:Meth. Enzimol, Academic Press, New York, v. 52C, p. 302-310, 1977.

127. SEDLAK, J.; LINDSAY, R.H. Estimation of total protein-bound, non-protein sulphydryl group in tissue with Ellman's reagent. Anal. Biochem., Orlando Fl., v. 25, p. 192-2O5, 1968.

128. TIETZE, F. Enzymatic method for quantitative determination of nanogram amounts of total and oxidized gluthatione: aplicatinos to mammalian blood and other tissues. Anal Biochem, Orlando

Fl., v. 27, p. 502-522, 1969.

129. GALLET, P.F.; MALTAH, A.; PETIT, J-M.; DENIS-GAY, M.; JULIEN, R. Direct cardiolopin assay in yeast using the red fluorescent emission of 10-N-nonyl acridine orange. Eur. J. Biochem., Berlin, New York, Springer, v. 228, p. 113-119, 1995.

130. PUMFORD, N. R.; HALMES, N.C.; HINDSON, J.A. Covalent binding of xenobiotics to specific proteins in the liver. Drug Metab Rev., New York, v. 29, n. 1&2, p. 39-57, 1997.

131. FARISS, M. W.; CHAN, C. B.; PATEL, M.; VAN HOUTEN, B. Role of mitochondria in toxic oxidative stress. Mol. Interv., Bethesda, v. 5, n. 2, p. 94-111, 2005.

132. GOEL, M.R.; SHARA, M.A.; STOHS, S.J. Induction of lipid peroxidation by hexlorocyclohexezene, dieldrin, TCDD, carbon tetrachoride, and hexachlorobenzene in rats. Bull Environ Contam Toxicol., Springer Verlag, v. 40, p. 255-62, 1988.

133. KALGUTKAR, A.S.; OBACH, R.S.; MAURER, T.S. Mechanism-based inactivation of cytochrome P450 enzymes: chemical mechanisms, structure-activity relationships and relationship to clinical drug-drug interactions and idiosyncratic adverse drug reactions. Curr Drug Metab., Hilversum, Netherlands, v. 5, p. 407-47, 2007.

134. TOMPKINS, L.M.; WALLACE, A.D. Mechanisms of cytochrome P450 induction. J Biochem Mol Toxicol., New York, NY, v. 21 n. 4, p. 176-81, 2007.

135. TONG, V.; TENG, X.W.; CHANG, T.K.; ABBOTT, F.S. Valproic acid II: effects on oxidative stress, mitochondrial membrane potential, and cytotoxicity in glutathione-depleted rat hepatocytes. Toxicological Sciences, Orlando, FL, v. 86, p. 436-43, 2005.

136. BOELSTERLI, U.A.; LIM, P.L. Mitochondrial abnormalities--a link to idiosyncratic drug hepatotoxicity? Toxicology and Applied Pharmacology, New York, v. 220, p. 92-107, 2007.

137. FLORA, S.J. Role of free radicals and antioxidants in health and disease. Cell Mol Biol, (Noisy-le-grand), Oxford ; Elmsford, N. Y., v. 53, n. 1, p. 1-2, 2007.

138. VALKO, M.; LEIBFRITZ, D.; MONCOL, J.; CRONIN, M.T.; MAZUR, M.; TELSER, J. Free radicals and antioxidants in normal physiological functions and human disease. Int J Biochem Cell Biol., Pergamon, v. 39, n. 1, p. 44-84, 2007.

139. DRIEFUS, F.E.; LANGER, D.H. Hepatic considerations in the use of antiepileptic drugs. Epilepsia, New York, v. 28 (Suppl. 2), p. S23-29, 1987.

140. DWIVEDI, R.; GOGTAY, N.; KHARKAR, V.; AMLADI, S.; KSHIRSAGAR, N. In- vitro lymphocyte toxicity to a phenytoin metabolite in phenytoin induced cutaneous adverse drug eruptions. Indian Journal of Dermatology, Venereology and Leprology, Vellore, v. 70, p. 217-20,

2004.

141. KALAPOS, M.P. Carbamazepine-provoked hepatotoxicity and possible aetiopathological role of glutathione in the events. Retrospective review of old data and call for new investigation. Adverse Drug Reactions and Toxicological Reviews, Oxford, v. 21, p. 123141, 2002

142. HAUKELAND, J.W.; JAHNSEN, J.; RAKNERUD, N. Carbamazepine-induced hepatitis. Tidsskrift for den Norske Laegeforening, Oslo, v. 120, p. 2875-2877, 2000.

143. COON, K.D.; VALLA, J.; SZELINGER, S.; SCHNEIDER, L.E.; NIEDZIELKO, T.L.; BROWN, K.M.; PEARSON, J.V.; HALPERIN, R.; DUNCKLEY, T.; PAPASSOTIROPOULOS, A.; CASELLI, R.J.; REIMAN, E.M.; STEPHAN, D.A. Quantitation of heteroplasmy of mtDNA sequence variants identified in a population of AD patients and controls by array-based resequencing. Mitochondrion v. 6, p. 194-210, 2006.

144. HOCH, F.L. Cardiolipins and biomembrane fuction. Biochim. Biophys. Acta, Amsterdam, v. 1113, p. 71-133, 1992.

145. BERNARDI, P. The permeability transition pore. Control points of a cyclosporin Asensitive mitochondrial channel involved in cell death. Biochim. Biophys. Acta, Amsterdam, v. 1275, p. 5-9, 1996.

146. CASTILHO, R.F.; KOWALTOWSKI, A.J.; MEINICKE, A.R.; BECHARA, E.J.; VERCESI, A.E., Permeabilization of the inner mitochondrial membrane by Ca2+ ions is stimulated by t-butyl hydroperoxide and mediated by reactive oxygen species generated by mitochondria. Free Radic Biol Med. New York, v. 18, n. 3, p. 479-86, 1995.

147. VERCESI, A.E. Ca transport and oxidative damage of mitochondria. Braz. J. Med. Res., Sao Paulo, v. 26, p. 441-457, 1993.

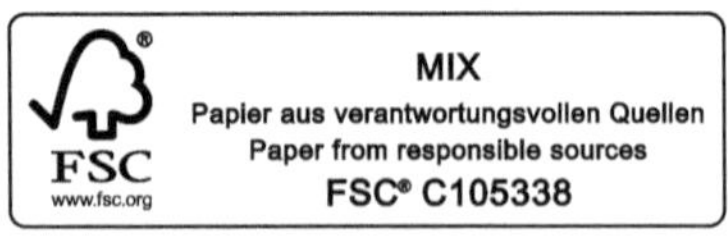

Printed by Books on Demand GmbH, Norderstedt / Germany